214 600

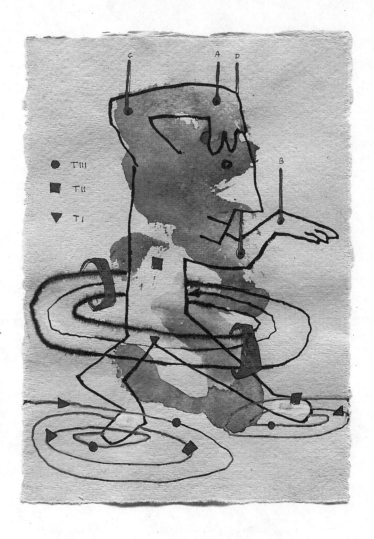

THE ART OF THE STRAIGHT LINE

LOU REED

THE ART OF THE STRAIGHT LINE

MY TAI CHI

Edited by
Laurie Anderson
Stephan Berwick
Bob Currie
and Scott Richman

A collection of
Lou's writing on Tai Chi
and conversations
with friends, teachers, and
fellow practitioners

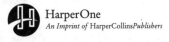

HarperOne
An Imprint of HarperCollins Publishers

Page 7: "I'll Be Your Mirror" lyrics by Lou Reed, reprinted with permission of Hal Leonard LLC. Pages 43, 101, 131, and 167: Excerpts from "Lou Reed: The Taiji Raven Speaks" by Martha Burr, *Kung Fu Tai Chi* magazine, May/June 2003, reprinted with permission of Gene Ching, *Kung Fu* magazine. Page 43: Excerpt from interview for Rock On, BBC Radio 1, March 26, 1983, reprinted with permission of the BBC. Page 102: Excerpt from interview by Rob Hogendoorn for "Brainwave: Sacred Science," Rubin Museum of Art, January 30, 2008, reprinted with permission of Rubin Museum. Pages 136–39: Excerpt from "Lou Reed: A Walk on the Wild Side of Tai Chi" by Martha Burr, *Kung Fu Tai Chi* magazine, May/June 2003, reprinted with permission of Gene Ching, *Kung Fu* magazine. Pages 139–40: Excerpt from interview for *We Talk*, SinoVision, 2011, reprinted with permission of Stella Gu. Pages 168–71: Excerpt from "Lou Reed on Tai Chi" by Gene Ching, *Kung Fu Tai Chi* magazine, June 2012, reprinted with permission of Gene Ching, *Kung Fu* magazine. Pages 172–73: Excerpt from interview by Bob Belinoff, "Sitting Down with Lou Reed: On Tai Chi, Meditation Music, and Care of the Knees," *LA Yoga* magazine, June 2007, reprinted with permission of *LA Yoga*. Pages 174–76: Excerpt from interview by Liz Belilovskaya, "Mass Destruction: Lou Reed and Stephan Berwick Talk *Final Weapon*," Planet III, April 2012, reprinted with permission of Liz Belilovskaya. Pages 184–85: "New Scar Right Over My Heart" by Anne Waldman, reprinted with permission of Anne Waldman. Page 306: "The Power of the Heart" lyrics by Lou Reed, reprinted with permission of Hal Leonard LLC.

HarperCollins books may be purchased for educational, business, or sales promotional use. For information, please email the Special Markets Department at SPsales@harpercollins.com.

FIRST EDITION

Designed by Yolanda Cuomo

Associate designer: Bobbie Richardson

Library of Congress Cataloging-in-Publication Data has been applied for.

ISBN 978-0-06-309353-9

23 24 25 26 27 TC 10 9 8 7 6 5 4 3 2 1

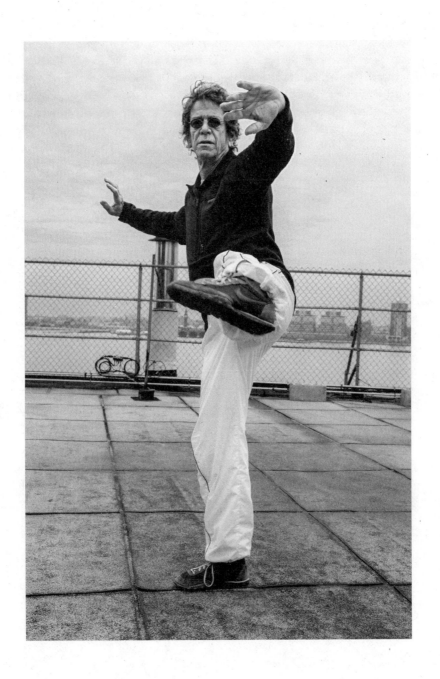

CONTENTS

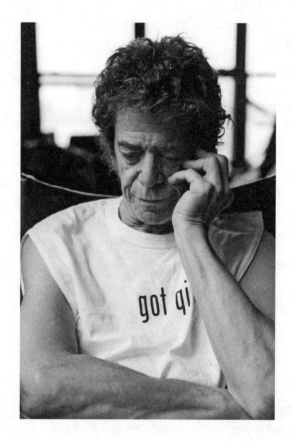

Lou on the phone

MY TAI CHI

Over the years I've been asked: How do you stay in shape? How do you take care of your back? Knees? Various joints that start to lose their elasticity as we age? The answer? The Four Noble Truths—there is suffering, the cause of suffering, the end of suffering, and the path that leads to the end of suffering.

So life is suffering. We all age. We all know it. We watch our parents, our friends wither, struck down by time. I watched my cousin Shirley, at 102, endure this. She said it was too much. She wished it was over. I asked her what her secret was to deal with the endless pain, the hospitals, the inability to see—macular degeneration. Her mind so sharp, she said, "What can you do?" This was her particular wisdom.

People ask about getting old because they know I probably shouldn't be here—a study in reckless excess. Yet here I am, and at age sixty-eight.

I have studied Tai Chi for more than twenty-five years. The first fifteen or so in preparation for my adventures with my teacher Master Ren GuangYi.

I had seen a video of Master Ren. So I went to see him in his rented dance studio opposite the Public Theater. Anyone who has seen him and has interest in the art becomes his student. We all do. I wanted to learn his technique of explosive internal power: fajin. I study six to seven days a week for two hours a day when not touring. I've done demos with Master Ren everywhere from Carnegie Hall to the steps of the Sydney Opera House, where we did a seminar this past spring.

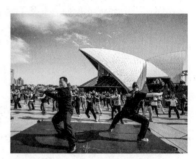

When I tour, it is with my Tai Chi. Not to get too flowery here, but I want more out of life than a gold record and fame. I want to mature like a warrior. I want the power and grace I never had a chance

Tai Chi lessons and demonstrations at Vivid Festival in Sydney, Australia, 2010, curated by Lou and Laurie

to learn. Master Ren's teacher Chen Xiaowang told me that the Tai Chi would protect me. How?

Because Tai Chi puts you in touch with the invisible power of—yes—the universe. The best of energies become available, and soon your body and mind become an invisible power. My Tai Chi has protected my body. Change your energy; change your mind. You have more ability than you know. The unexamined life and all that.

You don't need equipment. My teacher has made forms (a series of choreographed moves) that can be done in an apartment with very little space. They are called compact.

I do not want to go gently into fat-senility-lethargy. We can do better than that, although our culture makes it difficult. (Other countries teach art or meditation in school. We have woodshop. Life for the uninspired.) Tai Chi is also a martial art of unparalleled sophistication. It is a system put together to maintain health and physical prowess.

Master Ren was a heavyweight champion of Chinese boxing [Tai Chi Chuan]. He is a great artist and teacher. His Tai Chi should be taught in universities, public schools, and hospitals. It is life-changing. All the same, you must have an authentic instructor. To correct alignment and save and strengthen the knees and back. The story of Master Ren is one for a film. Perhaps another time.

I wish I could convince you to change your life and save your body and soul. I know it sounds too good. But truly: Tai Chi—why not?

—LOU REED, FROM THE ORIGINAL LETTER PUBLISHED
BY THE *NEW YORK TIMES*, OCTOBER 26, 2010

Lou's notes for the book, 2009

WHOLE BODY IS ONE BIG TENDON.

"THE ART OF THE STRAIGHT LINE"
"THE ART OF TAI CHI"
    SHOULDER TIP ELBOW TIP FIST TIP
    POWER GOES FROM MIND THRU TO TIP.

<u>INTRO</u> : DR. DAN RICHMAN

"CUT ENERGY" LIKE KNIFE
LIKE CAT / "READY"

GUEST APPEARANCE

任
廣
義

<u>REN</u>

GUANGYI REN

Ren, GY   REN GUY
    G. Y

REN GY   REN G.Y.

REN GY   REN GYE

     REN GYI

任 方è

REN, G.Y 太极

REN, GUANGYI   REN GEE

FOREWORD

The title *The Art of the Straight Line* is pure Lou. Tai Chi is made of circles, circles within circles. So what's straight? Well, that's the art! How to move through circles without losing your sense of direction and your overall goal.

Lou loved to talk about Tai Chi, and he was an enthusiastic teacher. He was excited about writing this book, and he started out with lots of ideas and plans. But too many things intervened, and the book he began in 2009 was left as scattered notes when he died in 2013.

At the beginning of the project, we named ourselves the Eds. We come from very different worlds. Scott Richman worked and traveled with Lou, Bob Currie spent time with him as a friend, Stephan Berwick—a Chinese-style martial artist and writer—was also a friend of Lou's, and I was his partner for twenty-one years. Together, we set out to put this book together.

Fortunately, Lou had many fellow Tai Chi practitioners and friends. In addition to Lou's own words, their voices and varied perspectives add to the richness and depth of this document. Me, I've learned a lot from the people we interviewed. As editors, we were struck by how many of them felt especially close to him. He was many people's best friend. One of Lou's most transcendent songs was "I'll Be Your Mirror." Observing, understanding, and empathizing with people were among his greatest skills.

I'll be your mirror. Reflect what you are.

in case you don't know.

I'll be the wind, the rain and the sunset.

The light on your door to show that you're home.

We didn't plan to talk with a lot of people, but each interview added another note to what became a multifaceted portrait. In the end, Lou is the true author of this book. We see it as a helpful and specific "how-to" as well as an exciting picture of a side of Lou that few people know.

Lou wanted to write a book that would inspire people to learn about and do Tai Chi. He often showed people moves, corrected their posture, and gave advice about how to move. We all miss his voice—hilarious and dead serious at once. As the author, he would be addressing you as directly as possible. We hope this collection conveys the urgency, commitment, and sense of humor in his voice and that as the book unfolds you will find a way into this deep practice.

—LAURIE ANDERSON

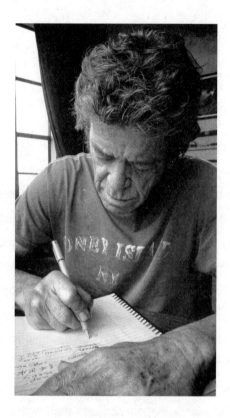

Lou making notes on Tai Chi forms

A. M. HOMES

Author and creative-writing professor at Princeton University

SCOTT RICHMAN: The work started on this book in 2009. Lou had a tough time getting it off the ground and then he asked for your help. We have that email.

STEPHAN BERWICK: That email of yours actually helped us out a lot.

A. M. HOMES: Lou and I often talked about creative processes—how do you do something or how do you make something. But I also had no idea what I said to him. If I remember anything, it was about him having questions about how to structure things, how to shape it, and where to begin. He talked to me about Tai Chi, and oh, it sounds too enormous to say. It saved him. It was really central to his sense of well-being, self-regulation, a sense of a place to go explore. I think he found literally strength and energy and calm in it. He also liked to turn other people on to it. Just getting somebody excited about it meant an enormous amount to him. And he loved going to class, and he loved the range of people who were in the class. It was, like, at the core of where his investment was. And he asked for my advice about how to write this.

LAURIE ANDERSON: Could you read the email you sent to Lou?

A. M.: Okay. "Notes for Lou. Teacher, think of questions. Do a full detailed interview. Re: how he manages health, his own emotions, his powers. Other students, what the practice means to them, their biographies, how they got to this point. Write about, ask about. Teacher is mentor. Flaws. Why teach?

What does it mean to pass it on? Focus, a mastery of energy, how the practice teaches you when to expand and when to contract, how that also applies to decision making, anger management, the practice's habit, the progression over time, how the person changes, and how the practice changes."

LAURIE: We're following your outline as well as we can.

A. M.: I know. [*Continues reading email.*] "Lou, use your own words. Act like a slow-motion camera. Use your language to describe the learning. Think of it as a long poem or lyric. I've told you a million times, just remember today. Physically and aesthetically thrilling, it could change your life. Detail how. Make a list of twenty things without stopping to think. And if you keep doing it, it just starts to happen. What does it mean to be ready to fight? To hold great power in reserve? Sitting, you can't sit like this, you're not ready." Lou also would talk a lot about positions. And he would just reach over sometimes and shove you. Just to knock you over! To show you that you just were not ready. I mean . . . really? That's what that note is about.

[*Continues reading email.*] "Lou, your biography, your personal history of the practice. When did you start? Where were you? What was your life like at the time? Where did you first go to practice? Early teachers. What did you learn? Did you stop and start? How did you take it with you on the road? How your life changed. How you've changed." And then there's a quote [from Lou in reply]: "I like martial arts people. They're straightforward. You know they went through it too. You watch out for wise guys—when the guys have shown you something, they hurt you."

He was very aware of that too. Of the way people could physically hurt each other and the stupidity in it. The stupidity in doing the move to show off, overreaching one's own boundary. And he would look at you and laugh. "I could kill you. But I'm just choosing not to in this moment."

Lou had an incredible sense of humor; in the midst of a very serious thing, he would just crack up. Which I think makes him different [from] a lot of other Tai Chi practitioners, because they're not always laughing. He took himself seriously, but there was always that crack that you could just cleave open for a good joke. Anyway, he said [in reply], "Put in practice, because of power and confidence. People who pick up on it can't knock me down."

[*Continues reading email.*] "Sections of your story, your teacher's story. Think of ten or fifteen questions to ask, the same questions for each person. Ask them, 'What is the secret you're not willing to tell me? The thing you fear most? What drives you?' Open questions about life, focus, desire, mastery. How you get what you want. Learning to operate and to trust one's intuition." And then there's, "Look at Lou Reed not shaking now. Contrast between who you were and who you've become. Your own personal journey." And then there's this big blank page that Lou didn't fill out [reply to].

When we talked about Tai Chi, we talked about the sense of mastery and control, and I always felt that when Lou talked about it, it was a place where he felt very in himself. And it sort of allowed him to navigate other things that he would not have navigated as gracefully.

He was always saying, "Try to come to class. Come with me. Come with me and Ren. Come do this. You have to do that. You're gonna die if you don't." It was always now. It was not later.

And also, we'd go on pizza adventures. You know, you had to go far for pizza. Or there would be that one pizza place in the East Village that only bakes till they run out of whatever.

LAURIE: You know, one of the moves in the Chen Tai Chi 19 Form—such a beautiful move—he named Delivering the Pizza, and it really looked like that: one arm, palm up, like a cartoon chef carrying a hot pie. And the name made it easier for people to remember the move.

A. M.: It's funny, as Lou got older, he got to be a foodie. And when I met him, he was going out to Barolo places with Oscar Hijuelos. My sense of Oscar always was that Oscar was sort of complicated, very playful, and also melancholy. And I think he and Lou understood that part of each other. The playful sparring, and then with this other layer of something.

LAURIE: And they loved watching boxing together and smoking cigars, and then they would eventually move to playing slow, sad things on their guitars.

Why do you think he didn't write this book?

A. M.: I think it's the difficulty of it. And it's funny, because it's what he did in his songs all the time. But it was the difficulty of combining the incredibly, deeply cellularly personal ideas into words. Not just personal in the most physical sense of it but with a kind of larger, philosophical spiritual idea. And it was hard to render that in language with structure. I think it seemed difficult to him because it was a truly felt thing.

LAURIE: Did you see Tai Chi in his writing?

A. M.: Sometimes, in his sense of movement or rhythm and the ability to be both abrupt and not.

STEPHAN: We used to say to him, "Why don't you just use the dictation app on the phone and just start talking into it?" And even that was hard.

A. M.: It's not that kind of language. How do you create the language of talking about this and how would Lou create Lou's language of Tai Chi out of not just the physical movements of it but a verbal, a spoken language of Tai Chi? That would be something I'd wanna ask him.

SCOTT (on listening to Lou's voice at an event the night before the interview): When Lou verbalized some of the concepts of Tai Chi that we got from the commentary, we isolated that stuff. But it was part of the discussion, of working something out as a group.

A. M.: And I have to say, when I was listening, I didn't want to look up. I just want to hear Lou across the room. I just want to be standing here while he's talking over there. That sort of thing. He sounded young and strong and, like, you know?

LAURIE: You forget that he had plenty of ups and downs in the last bit of his life, times when he was very strong again. And he talks to us from the afterworld.

A. M.: I hate when that happens, but I think he's receptive to the . . . you know!

LAURIE: Lou used to use the Ouija board all the time. So what would you ask if there was a Ouija board?

A. M.: I think I could picture a whole different kind of sound coming out of Lou. What is the verbal sound of Tai Chi? What is the language?

LAURIE: He did that in music. And Ren and Lou did a lot of drawings together—diagrams of how Tai Chi works. That's probably the closest to language that that came.

Back to the Ouija board. What would you ask Lou right now? He's been gone over five years.

A. M.: I would ask him what he's been working on. I was thinking about, when you were just showing me those drawings, about lab notation and the way choreographers mark their dances—their specific language. It was Doris Humphrey who came up with the system of that. But what is the language of that? How do you show the flow?

BOB CURRIE: That was a failed language, though. Because they only showed the front.

LAURIE: Well, in Tai Chi **Push Hands** training you watch it, you almost see the flow of chi. If you start visualizing it, you can see how it moves down your shoulder and then up your arm and then into someone else's and back. You start to see

PUSH HANDS, or "Tui Shou," is partner training in Tai Chi.

energy flow. And Lou was saying something last night in the last part of the recording about how he had his head coming in and out of focus. And he talked about how everyone is so individual. He makes that really clear.

SCOTT: Everyone expresses their energy differently.

LAURIE: Something like that. Yeah. It really jumped out for me, because it wasn't somebody pontificating about chi.

SCOTT: He really did express it through language when he was talking with other people. And his guitar sounds made me feel the chi. When he did stuff like that, you really felt it.

A. M.: But is it because it articulated some of the shifts?

LAURIE: Each note called attention to itself in that way. Yeah. It had this gnarl. Or, like you said, they weren't polite.

STEPHAN: There was something a little bit provocative about it. And then it kind of ignites something in people.

A. M.: Lou totally got that everybody had their own energy. And there were people that other people didn't like and Lou liked them. And he liked them even if their energy was super complicated. He liked them for who they were. And even, for lack of a better word, for their commitment to themselves.

LAURIE: The other thing about it was his just straight-up generosity. We would go to shows and films and concerts almost every night, and he would always find something good about them, and I would often find something negative.

A. M.: Right. Right. But see, there's something about that, that to me was always so interesting, because on the one hand, he could be so cranky. And then, on the other hand, this incredible optimist.

But back to Tai Chi: the physicality of it gave him both physical strength but also a spiritual or creative expansion. I can remember seeing

Lou in shorts and his arms out a lot! There was the public Lou with sun-glasses, but for me Lou was mostly, I don't know, just regular Lou.

When my daughter, Juliet, was really little, she used to say, "Lou, I wanna go here." And Lou would do whatever Juliet said. And when we'd go to a restaurant and she would say, "I wish Lou were here, because then he would have gotten us a . . ." You know? But the funny thing was, there was this time when she had written a play on the death of Lincoln. And one of the kids who was supposed to play Lincoln bowed out, because she was afraid that after she died, the kids had to carry her away and they might drop her. And Lou said, "Well, I'll come and be Lincoln." And I remember we were all thinking, *That would be really funny. Lou Reed—for one night only—as Abe Lincoln in fourth grade!* But that was very Lou-like. "I'll just show up and, like, be Lincoln for an hour!" You know? It would have been great. Especially after one of the other actors, Mrs. Lincoln, ran off crying and I had to step in for Mrs. Lincoln. But yeah, I just, like, miss him, you know?

LAURIE: Isn't that weird? He's been gone for over five years.

A. M.: It doesn't seem like that. Honestly, I feel like we're just waiting. Like we're waiting for Lou to come back. I like hearing his voice a lot. I still have some messages on my machine.

STEPHAN: When he first started the book idea, he said *Zen in the Art of Archery* was something that inspired him.

A. M.: It's a book about creative and spiritual risk-taking.

LAURIE: And also targets. Because he had a goal. It's about how to get from here to there in this really circular structure!

SCOTT: Everyone's straight line is different.

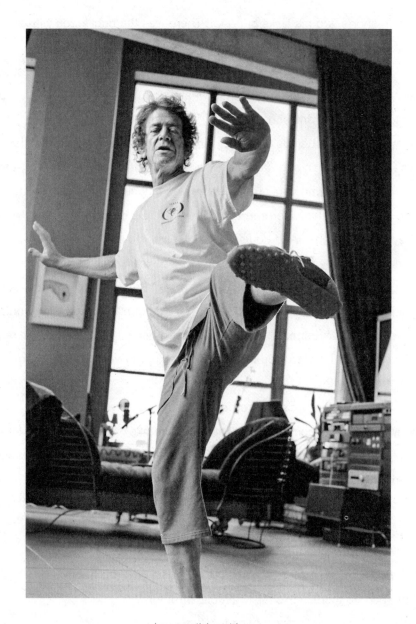

Lou practicing at home

CHAPTER 1

WHAT IS TAI CHI?

The Chinese say you meet the hard with the soft, the yin
with the yang, the down with the up

I have often thought of Tai Chi as some kind of physical unity to the universe itself, some strange ancient methodology that could link us to the basic energy wave of existence. I don't want to seem mystical, but something does happen to you when you practice this ancient art. There are history books about the families, the creators of all this, should you like to know. My concern is how it relates to myself and my classmates, who have all gone through the pain and practice of approaching the art. And it is an art, though rarely seen by us here in the States. It won't really help to see martial arts movies, as they will not show you. We are talking of the art and internal power of Tai Chi. Many people talk of internal power but they never actually do it. It's always some form of external force, like Bruce Lee's one-inch punch. I'm talking about no-inch punch. And not only punch but every part of your body—your chest, your elbow, your butt, your entire body at any time and any place.

Tai Chi frees you from preconceptions—music or tempo, this, that, or the other thing. It is, I think, a pretty enabling kind of thing. I hate to use that word, "enabling," but there it is. It's very, very useful for centering yourself, for experiencing these different kinds of disciplines, be it meditation, body-work, Tai Chi, Yoga, whatever. Or I like to just have it going all the time because it makes the outside sounds into a more musical environment.

—FROM LOU'S NOTES ON TAI CHI

TONY VISCONTI

Rock music producer and Tai Chi practitioner

I always loved martial arts. I wanted to learn how to defend myself. In the sixth grade, I had this fantastic teacher Mr. Flanagan. He talked about serving in World War II and said, "When I was in Asia, I saw a man who could break wood with his bare hands." I'm twelve years old and said to myself, "I have to learn how to break wood with my bare hands." My dad was a carpenter, so I started immediately with that. He had wood!

I started studying Tai Chi in 1980 with a teacher named John Kells, who later became a grandmaster. He studied Yang Tai Chi in Taiwan with a Dr. Chi Chiang-tao who was a Tai Chi master and a top student of Cheng Man-ch'ing. His whole thing was softness. You could rush him, you could try to punch him, grab him, then he'd barely touch you and you went flying through the air and ended up on the ground. This was uprooting power. His emphasized softness and relaxation for Push Hands. To this day I think of what he used to teach me if I become tense during practice. That was my beginning to Tai Chi, five years studying the Yang style with Grandmaster John Kells.

I met Lou back when he was making *Transformer* with David Bowie and he was kind of half sleeping on the studio floor. David was in proper Ziggy regalia. I couldn't see Lou anywhere until David said, "Oh, Tony, you should meet Lou. There he is." So I walked up to him with, "Hi, Lou." He looked up. "Hi, Tony." And he went back to sleep. That was the first time I met Lou, the very first time, in the '70s. After that, I would meet Lou with David in New York, but we never really talked much.

I went to lots of music biz events where Lou could be very hard-ass in person. Several times I'd bump into Lou but he just wouldn't acknowledge me, or maybe he'd forgotten that he'd met me. This was before we studied Tai Chi together. All those barriers melted away with Tai Chi. I think Lou worked out most of his anger around his early days of Tai Chi. You can't really be angry in martial arts. You can't afford that luxury. And that's something you learn quickly, depending on your teacher.

I reconnected with Lou in 2003. I was making an album with Bowie called *Reality*. David asked, "Are you still keeping up with your Tai

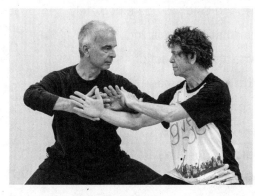

Chi?" I said, "Yeah, but I never found a teacher in New York that I liked." I wandered out to a few schools downtown, but they looked a little prohibitive. I could see that the teachers were masters but I could see the students, especially the non-Chinese people, didn't look good. I didn't know if they were being taught correctly or they

Tony and Lou doing Push Hands

just weren't good students. There was always a saying that Kung Fu teachers don't teach you "everything" just in case a student tries to take over the class.

In London I heard about Chen Tai Chi but couldn't find a book on it. Later, I saw a Tai Chi book that had a picture of a Chen master. The book had a brief description of the Chen style. I read that they'd leap, do jump kicks, which according to my Yang Tai Chi teacher, Grandmaster Kells, was wrong—your feet should never leave the ground, he'd say it wasn't Tai Chi. That was his own specific view of what Tai Chi should be; that it should be slow, meditative, it should be peaceful and non-aggressive.

Bowie suggested, "Why don't you speak to Lou. He seems to be quite into Tai Chi." Later on the phone Lou said, "Yeah, Tony, you've got to come down to a class." He said, "This guy is the real deal." And I went, because I knew Grandmaster Kells was also a real deal. I knew a real deal when I saw one. I watched a class. Lou wasn't there on that night. I watched Master Ren and I just fell in love with him. Master Ren was so confident, and he had a good open attitude. He also had a good sense of humor.

Master Ren said to me, "Oh, you're a friend of Lou?" And I said, "Yeah, that's right." He was expecting me, and I signed up immediately afterwards. I saw that the Chen style was what I was missing. With my background in other martial arts, I needed a little more action than Yang Tai Chi could provide. The leaps and explosive energy made sense when I saw Master Ren do the forms. I never forgot the lessons I learned in Yang, but I prefer Chen style because it gives me a workout and more information about how Tai Chi works. The lower postures are really good for me. I took to it immediately. And then it was lovely to see how advanced Lou was. He started before me. Lou said that his Eagle Claw teacher, Grandmaster Leung Shum, was also a Wu-style Tai Chi master. He once effortlessly threw Lou and Lou asked, "What was that?" Leung Shum said, "Tai Chi."

Joining Master Ren's group was a life-changer. After a ten-year search, I more or less gave up. After about a year of training, my legs became very strong. Ren always says, "You have two hearts. One is in your chest and the other is in your legs." But I felt weird sometimes because I studied a different style of Tai Chi. When I compared Chen to Yang styles I often became conflicted. During my first year with Master Ren, I had to undo a lot of my opinions, ideas—basically the chip on my shoulder. Grandmaster Kells always said, there's always a "door" if your wrist is grabbed, there's a "door" out. You're never completely trapped if you know how to unlock the "door." But when Master Ren first gripped me and put me in a lock, I thought, *Where the hell is this door that Kells spoke about?* I was in agony. But that was a rite of passage all the students had to go through—you had to feel the power of Chen Tai Chi. Funnily, when Master Ren asked for a volunteer to give a demonstration of this power, you could see several students clearly take a step or two backwards.

The Tai Chi hand is rounded and relaxed, its natural state. Also I learned that chi does not travel through a tense body. The body and mind have to be relaxed, not floppy, but in the Yin mode. The muscles have to be relaxed for the chi to flow. This is where your awareness to internal strength begins. You learn how to undo layers of tension in order to find strength from a deeper source.

I also studied the Alexander Technique. The basic principles of Tai Chi and the Alexander Technique are almost one and the same. You don't go against the grain. Body parts and limbs bend in a certain way, in harmony with natural lines of energy. I suffered from sciatica a lot of my early adult life, but during my Tai Chi form practice the pain left me. I had two physical lives. One was when I did Tai Chi. I was relaxed. I was in harmony. I was doing everything right. And then I would do something stupid and injure my lower back or neck. I'd been to chiropractors, osteopaths, acupuncturists, etcetera. One day I was browsing in Foyles Bookshop in London. A book fell off the bargain table right on my foot! It was a book on the Alexander Technique. I read in the first pages that inherently humans don't have bad backs or necks. But wear and tear of unconscious actions makes you injure yourself. The first thing you learn in an Alexander Technique lesson is that you never knew how to sit and stand properly. After time your tortured body makes most people in pain go to a doctor for pills. That made total sense after I hurt my back when my wife handed me our infant son across the table in a restaurant, and I bent way over the table to pick him up. He weighed about twelve pounds. And my back went *ping*, and sent a sharp pain down my sciatic nerve. I had bad weeks periodically when climbing out of bed took twenty minutes or more because of sciatica.

I wasn't applying Tai Chi to my normal life. I was being irresponsible and unconscious in my day-to-day life. After my first five or so Alexander lessons I understood. Eureka! It's the same principle in Tai Chi (moving the head up to heaven and the feet firmly on the ground). F. M. Alexander discovered Tai Chi principles on his own in isolated Tasmania, in the early twentieth century, as an actor who was often in pain. My Tai Chi and my Alexander Technique improved my well-being when I put both practices together.

Tai Chi is beautiful in that it has three benefits. It's got the health benefits. You practice the forms slowly to strengthen your body and also to give your internal organs a kind of massage. The second thing, which is equally important, it's a form of meditation. Lou and I were attracted to this. Your mind becomes tranquil, very relaxed. The Standing Mountain pose helps you to scan your body for tension and tells it to relax. Number three is you learn how to defend yourself. That may not be important to everyone, but it's there. It's built in. The self-defense applications are harder to learn than Karate and such external styles, so most people who begin Tai Chi aren't even aware it's a martial art because it is practiced slowly. Of course, a Tai Chi expert such as our Master Ren moves at lightning speed if he were to defend himself. It is not necessary to learn the self-defense part of Tai Chi to get the health and meditative benefits.

We used to train in Master Ren's class to traditional Chinese music softly in the background. One day Ren comes

STANDING MOUNTAIN, or Standing Post, is the basic standing exercise used to build one's correct structural strength and optimize energy flow.

in with a cassette for the class boom box and says, "Lou wrote something for us." I felt, *Oh my God. What's this going to be?* It turned out to be an hour-long deep drone played on a synthesizer, with wavy, swooshy tone shaping. When I first heard it, I was on the fence about it. Someone actually never returned to class after they heard that! It was not that traditional thing! Eventually, I saw that it came from Lou's heart and from his earnest study of Tai Chi. And I should have known better. We've been practicing in class to Lou's music for several years now.

Master Ren onstage with Lou was just the most eye-opening thing. He performed the Chen Broadsword form to Lou's "The Raven." I'm sure more than a few people began Tai Chi practice after seeing them together onstage.

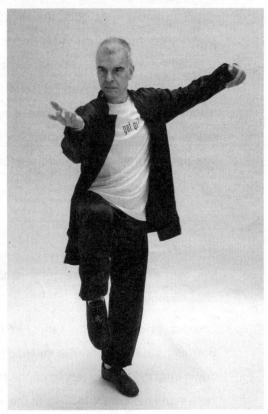

Lou and I trained together so much. We did intense seminars together with Grandmaster Chen Xiaowang and Master Chen Ziqiang visiting from Chen Village in China. Lou was often my training partner. Together in class we would help each other with form and technique. Lou always wanted to teach and Master Ren recognized that quality in him. Often in the advanced classes, he would ask Lou to teach me the material I missed after months working abroad. Lou would patiently show

Tony Visconti

me what I had missed. Lou made himself available to others in our class too. He was a straight-up elder brother classmate and, even at lunch afterwards, he was just one of us.

We lived only a few blocks apart in the West Village and many times when I was doing Tai Chi on my roof, he was sometimes on his roof with Master Ren getting a private lesson. Ren would call my phone and say, "Lou and I are here on the roof. Wave," and I would, then Ren would wave his jacket back. Lou would say, "I can see Tony!" We were in sync. I never directly thanked Lou for bringing me into the class but he and I became firm Tai Chi brothers.

Lou and I lived quite the rock and roll life in the '60s and '70s. Discovering Tai Chi later in life helped both of us to heal and live longer, gave us extra years. A lot of people from our generation died before their time. Tai Chi is a lifesaver. Tai Chi practice every day will give you good health and "eureka" experiences, insight to a move you suddenly understand. My work as a record producer and musician has never been better due to daily practice of Tai Chi. It's the best high I've ever experienced in my whole life.

RAMUNTCHO MATTA

Musician, artist, Tai Chi practitioner, and founder of Lizières, centre de cultures et de ressources in France

Lou didn't remember, but I met him for the first time in '79 with William Burroughs in New York. The meeting was in a restaurant in Union Square, down from the Warhol studio on the right, facing the Warhol building. We were in the restaurant looking at the window, and William said, "You see, you can see the energy of people." And Lou said, "Of course."

That was quite a magic experience, because William learned that in Mexico and in Morocco, yet Lou felt exactly the same. They were a match. I reminded Lou of this later when he was doing a concert in Lyon and we spent a lot of time in the gyms of hotels. And I think to work on that aspect of Lou, it's true that you have to do detective work for the past. It's also detective work of the future.

One of our last discussions was in Paris, and Lou was crying because he was saying how stupid he was to spend so much time in his lifetime destroying himself instead of discovering what he was discovering and what he was touching.

That was in Paris in 2011. He wanted to come to Lizières. And we went to see Jean-François Masson, a homeopathic doctor. I wanted to bring Lou on my motorbike, but he refused. He said he was a biker himself and would never go on the back. He was too scared. We went there. He was very sick at that moment. I did all the translation for him.

Masson's first job was as a cancer doctor. Then he discovered how the medicine in the late '70s was destroying the body. So he went to spend two years in Mexico in the mountains to study shamanic techniques. And then he studied five years in China. He's still practicing. He would ask very weird questions, like what is the color of cold for you? What is the smell of sadness?

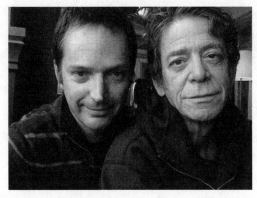
Ramuntcho Matta and Lou

I went with Lou to see Masson on three different trips to France. And the time I'm speaking to you about was the last trip. Lou was very sick. Usually, he was making a package for Lou with a lot of herbs and different things, etcetera. This time, he just gave him one little homeopathic thing, and it worked. He called me the day after, saying, "Wow, Ramuntcho, it's just amazing. I don't know what's inside this stupid little white thing, but I'm feeling a hundred percent better."

And he spent a lot of time crying. He knew that if he had spent less time destroying himself, he could have been in another level. And we argued a little bit because we don't have the same feeling about Tai Chi. He was still at the level of the fighting. And I'm more in the level of medicine.

Of course when we practiced, he was fighting because he loves to have fights. But one of the last sessions we had was a meditation one, and that was amazing, because he was really inside the energy in three seconds. I was always trying to take him somewhere else than fighting. I tried to bring him to the inside chi instead of the external one.

[*Laurie and Ramuntcho are in a car traveling to his Tai Chi/art/meditation center in Lizières outside Paris.*]

I did twelve years of Karate. And after, I did ten years of Aikido. And then I got paralyzed for three years after a long illness. That's why when I do Tai Chi, I do something different. I'm not saying I'm bionic. My two Tai Chi masters told me that I was learning very slow but in a very, very big way. And Lou was really interested in that.

KARATE AND AIKIDO are Japanese martial arts, based on older Chinese styles, that emerged in the early twentieth century.

One day I was practicing with a big, big, big master and he came to me—and we were fifty people working—he came to me and said, "Ramuntcho, you know you don't have to do Tai Chi like the others," and I said, "But why?" He said, "Because you're an artist. That means, when you're an artist you make something with your chi and you transmit your chi in your work, not by practicing. You do more Tai Chi in your work than most of the people who are doing Tai Chi." For me, that's the real lesson. That means we have to work.

You know Ramon Llull? He was a fourteenth-century Spanish mystic and mathematician. He made the wheel of fortune. For everything in life, you need a special wheel. A, B, C, D, E, F, G, H, I, J, K. Every time you want something in life, you have to have a relationship with two other things. Otherwise, it will never work. And it's very important for people to understand that if they have a goal, they have to work from the bottom up to build it. For example, you have to work your body because music without body won't work and what would be the third thing?

LAURIE ANDERSON: Well, if the body is the second, your heart is the third, I guess. Could it be all sorts of things?

RAMUNTCHO MATTA: Of course, but different sorts of things at different moments. But you have to think about that wheel all the time because you have to correspond. Otherwise, you get lost in the why. Lou was a Tai Chi guy too, but not only. He was out to transmit the essential. And the essential is not in the practice of the Tai Chi. It's in the enlightenment of the chi, which is an everyday life thing. [*They arrive at the center and begin to walk around.*]

So we have to really make an effort to remember. It's hard to find one string because everything is related. I remember a concert of the Velvet Underground in Paris. And I was in the balcony and I saw Lou was preparing to play. Within a few seconds everything changed. One moment there was Lou and the next there was Tai Chi. [*He demonstrates a shift in posture.*]

LAURIE: What you're showing us is somebody walking with his head and shoulders down and he suddenly focuses and stands straight.

RAMUNTCHO: It's not straight, it's relaxed and related. The related is very important because that's when you tune with another music. It has to do with that. I tried to do a church about Tai Chi. People who practice Tai

Chi say, "You have to practice Tai Chi." And for me, it's a little problem. It can let you fall into another compulsion. To practice five hours a day. To practice all the weapons. It can be an addiction too.

What Lou was doing with the chi is a very interesting point. He told me several times that Tai Chi was more important for him than music, and I said, "Yes, because now with Tai Chi you can do another music." And he said, "Oh yes, you're right." What I think is important about Lou and Tai Chi is to see that Tai Chi helps your life. In all the pictures that I received from you, Lou is doing Tai Chi. It's not Lou cooking, walking, writing. Lou in normal life.

For me, he was really the incarnation of chi. And it's interesting that he was a big master of Tai Chi. And when we practiced, we met in hotels. We were practicing, and he was trying all the time to fight because he had all this thing about fighting. And it was strange that a person at this level was still interested in fighting.

But I saw that he appreciated fighting. He loved it. I was using my Tai Chi to avoid the fight. So sometimes when we practiced, he'd be ready to kill me, and at that point I would just disappear and then he would be furious. He would say, "We have to make contact!" and I said, "Why? Why do we have to make contact? We're already in contact."

I think the form is a dance, it's cool, but to connect you don't need to make the form. You need three series of revelation. One is the feet, the other is the hands, and the other is the head. I can show it to you. I'm going to have some enemies because usually you don't do that. Do you wish to see it?

LAURIE: Of course!

RAMUNTCHO: The essence of my Tai Chi, if we speak about the subject, is no more tension, we've allowed it to flow. So if you want to fight, what is the key of fighting? It's time. So to be allowed to find the good time, to come before your instinct, you have to slow down. The only way to be fast is to slow down and Lou and I spoke a lot about that. So the more intense the fight is, the more you have to slow down. So, the boat is around. You can call it a boat, you can call it a light. And then it goes up to your legs, to your knees, to you. . . . Where your leg is attached to your body? Where is it, can you show it to me?

[*Laurie points to the hip.*] Okay, everybody does the same mistake. Where is the leg attached? Here. [*He points to his lower abdomen.*] So when you turn, the connection is here. That's the first thing. When you come down, you do it in all the directions. The full movement of Tai Chi is when you turn from inside to outside, you empty yourself. That's the movement. And after you do the opposite, but by stacking at the beginning. Stacking at the beginning, the little boat on the feet, and then you have to wait until the boat or the light will give the sensation, the physiological sensation, of something that's happening. But you have to practice that for years. And not more, you're not going to succeed more if you work ten hours a day rather than ten minutes a day. That's important too because some people will tell you, "You have to practice, you have to practice."

Then, you put your feet like that to mask this part of the feet and then this part. You know Lou's feet? He hated that exercise. Lou would say, "Okay, let's fight." And I'd say, "Wait, where is your weight?" Where do you put yourself? On the front of the feet or on the back of the feet? If you put all the weight on your toes, you fall forward. So go back and feel what is happening on the feet. Where is the weight usually? That's the first sensation that I had to work on when I got back on my feet after I was paralyzed. Just do this exercise five minutes a day for one month and you will see the difference of the connection.

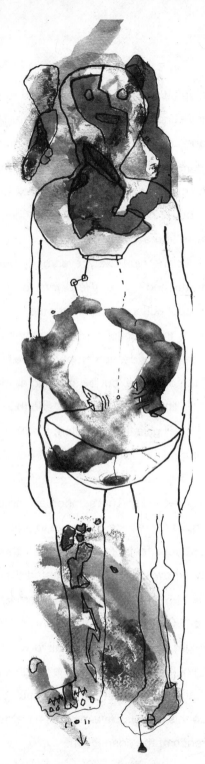

Portrait of Lou *by Ramuntcho Matta, watercolor, 2016*

You made that song with the words "people are in their bodies the way they drive in their cars." Remember? They know less about their bodies than their cars.

So now the hands. [*Points to his wrist.*] You know, what do you call that in English? What is the space you have between your wrist and your hand?

LAURIE: We don't have a name for it.

RAMUNTCHO: You have a space or not? So, first, you just do like that. [*Puts his palms together leaving an inch between them.*] The idea is not to go far, you know? To have a little light in between the two. And then you put one hand to the ground and the other hand to the sky. Can you feel the difference in your palm between the hand to the ground and the feeling of the stars in your hands? Can you feel the difference?

LAURIE: Yes.

RAMUNTCHO: What's coming from Earth? What's coming from the sky? It can be interesting to work with that. And then, next time you do this, you lift and you do with your little finger, you lift the universe. And you see if you have any tension and now to avoid the tension is to move your whole body and you'll do that for all the fingers. The more you do it sweetly, the more it works.

And then you put your arms at your sides and forget your body and you just think back to your little boat, to the feet. And move just one finger. Just one finger. This is impossible to translate in your book. Impossible! It's an experiential experience, as you said before. After doing that with all fingers, you will have hands again. And then you can do the work that Lou loved. It's a magnetic fan, so in doing that exercise you amplify your polarity and you can really work — which is important.

It's difficult to say that in a few minutes, but if you take the time, you can practice. And then there's your head. What's happening with your head? You have to imagine a pencil that you put on the end of your

Put one hand to the ground and the other hand to the sky. Can you feel the difference in your palm between the hand to the ground and the feeling of the stars in your hands?

▲

nose. You've done that exercise in your life or not? You put a pencil on your nose and you make a straight line with the pencil on your nose. And then you stop and do the opposite—you put a pencil on your back and you do a vertical line. And then, on each ear, vertical lines and then horizontal lines. The nose, on the back, and on the ears. And then you think of what holds your head. What is holding your head? Do you know what is holding your head?

Can you think you have a little wire here that's holding your head? Here! [*He taps the top of his head.*]

So you connect to this little wire, this little light, and now all of your skeleton is suspended to your head. Now you can walk, with that head. And that's another secret of fighting because if you're fighting like a stone, you can be like Rocky and it works, really hit the people, etcetera, but if you're held up by your head, when people hit you, you're just dancing. And then you have the flexibility to move and do whatever you want. Voilà! I don't know how you can translate that.

Do the exercise! Because it works.

And another important thing that we didn't speak about is that every time you change movement, or direction, it's like a tennis ball that you're sending up in the air and when the ball is on the top, it's already coming down but it's not coming down yet. So when you do a movement what-ever it is, you know the series, you have to go down. Go down slow. Like the ball it seems like it disappears, like it stops. But it's already going somewhere else.

But I really think that the bible of Lou, the real story, would be his normal. Without cooking, unfortunately. Did he like to do the dishes?

LAURIE: No. There's no dishes. That's the advantage of no cooking, no dishes. We went to restaurants. One of his great skills was talking to people in restaurants. And he would find what they needed and he would give it to them. He knew how to do that.

If you're held up by your head, when people hit you, you're just dancing.

▲

RAMUNTCHO: I remember that. It was amazing. Even in an autograph for a few minutes, it was that feeling exactly. And that's the chi. That's the connection. Okay. You know Earth?

LAURIE: Yes.

RAMUNTCHO: It's the little stone we're standing on. To stand on this planet you have to be kind of, I made the drawing out already, you saw the drawing, I made the drawing for you about Lou and Tai Chi. So it goes to your feet, your arms will connect to left and right, and your head will connect to the Earth to allow the energy to come down to the center Earth and to go back wherever you need it. You know?

You can call it chakra, you can call it dantien or whatever you want. But you have to have this connection with the arms and the legs. So, to open the canal you have to have feet. I should have worn better socks. Stupid.

It's difficult to show without experiencing it. But, basically you put one foot in front of the other and you imagine a little boat. You have a little boat, you have turned around your feet, from inside to outside. You know why? To have fun.

Let's not be too serious about serious subjects, right? So, you make a boat, turn around your feet, until the boat—the feet—move. Which is a verification of the mental and the feet. And what are we working here on that? What comes before instinct? You know? We speak about fact, you know, and we knew it was often like that. And what comes before intuition? What do you think comes before intuition?

LAURIE: Sensation?

RAMUNTCHO: No. Before intuition. Before instinct.

LAURIE: Before instinct? I would say sensation.

RAMUNTCHO: Well, I believe it's intention.

Lou and Bill O'Connor, his oldest martial arts friend, had extensive and detailed conversations about martial arts of all kinds both in person and in ongoing email exchanges.

On Oct 14, 2002, at 6:12 AM,

Lou, Yes, exploding power is better than just power. I do agree with you that it is more inclusive, and also believe that the exploding power is the goal of martial arts training. Actually prefer Sifu's word; i.e., rather than exploding, substitute shaking. Then the definition of Taijiquan might be: Taijiquan is a martial system that generates shaking power through silk reeling. Bill.

Sent: Monday, October 14, 2002 12:31 PM
Subject: Re: highwayman cloak and cape

Indeed. Also, Lin suggested that the first motion of the advisory board is to award each other honorary doctorates (after all the Institute is an educational institution). We can have an awards ceremony with capes and ceremonial swords. They have the four diamonds. We can be the five doctors of Tai Chi. Bill.

(SightingtheRifle) Date: November 2, 2015 at 8:13 PM

The arms in martial arts are actually double swords. The forward arm is on the same side as the forward foot. The back arm is on the same side as is the back foot. Arms and leg match. When confronting an opponent, the palms face the opponent in such a position as if to catch limbs of an opponent, if he tries to strike them towards you. Strikes are usually delivered by an opponent so hard and so fast that it is difficult to catch but also easy to deflect, provided the arms are held in the ready position. This position is to align the palms with the shoulders. The forward palm's hand is aligned with the shoulder on the side of the back leg, while the inside palm's hand is aligned with the shoulder on same side as is the forward leg. If one were then to place [the] ball of one's thumb against the depression where the collar bone touches the shoulder joint and then simply extend the arm out and then drop one's elbow at the point of the full extension that's the ready position since the thumb aligns with opposite shoulder; so the two thumbs will end up both in line in the center of the body, as if one were to be sighting along a rifle. In fact, the ready position is exactly that: Sighting the Rifle. Bill.

On Apr 25, 2015, at 1:01 PM, William O'Connor wrote:

Paris in the Spring! Yes, well this is all stuff that Lou and I talked about over the years; so, use whatever you believe might help with the book on Taijiquan. As far as I know, the Chen Taijiquan is the only exercise system where all four points of hips and shoulders are open. Aside from the martial aspect (all martial systems have validity or else they wouldn't exist), keeping the four points open allows the "qi" ["chi"] to circulate and therefore maintain health. The idea is to be as productive as possible for as long as possible and to prevent the onset of age decrepitude and dementia and to maintain physical strength and mental agility so necessary for creativity. Chen Tai Chi keeps one going.

From: William O'Connor
Subject: How the fist is made
Date: May 19, 2015

Different martial styles utilize differently shaped fists, but all martial styles utilize some sort of fist. The problem is that when punching with a bare fist with no protection most people will suffer fractures of the fingers and the wrist. This is because the fist is not tight enough. In order to make a tight fist, one has to start with the correct position of the thumb when the hand is open. Point forward with the palm open with the index finger. The thumb is now on the inside of the index finger when pointing. Start coiling the three other fingers beginning with the pinky finger, then ring finger, then middle finger; so that the three fingers, pinky, ring, middle are coiled in and touching the palm. Keep pointing with the index finger. This is the pistol grip. It is how pistols are held, and it comes from the sword grip. So, now there are three fingers coiled in and two fingers pointing, the index and the thumb. Now, instead of pointing forward with the index finger, point inward with the index finger at a right angle.

This aligns the index finger large knuckles with the knuckles of the other three fingers. Once the knuckles are aligned, coil the index finger to the palm so that it joins the three previous fingers already coiled. The final finger, which is called the hammer (the thumb), is then cocked, by having it cover the index finger, the middle finger and the ring finger (all three fingers, not two); three fingers. This cocking action of the thumb covering three fingers when bent into a fist, is called the "hammer fist." The fist feels like it is hammer. It's tight. Injuries occur because the fist is not tight enough. A loose fist occurs when the base of the thumb only covers two fingers (index and middle), but a proper fist covers three (index, middle and ring also).

at 11:37 PM, William O'Connor wrote:

Before I forget again, because it is directly related to music and why music is utilized as an accompaniment to performing a Tai Chi form, and it doesn't matter which system is practiced, Tai Chi works on concept of "listening behind." And that's simply shifting focus from the visual to the auditory whenever performing any form. Physically, it is tuning down the judgmental, critical, evaluating portion of the brain (dorsolateral pre-frontal cortex), to the creative portion of the brain (medial pre-frontal cortex), what marksmen or snipers call brain "T-Zone" (it's the third eye), an action which animals do naturally when confronted with novel situations: ears shift forward and up so they can take in more sound. This is the "listening behind" in Tai Chi. The focus is shifted from the dorsolateral pre-frontal cortex at the side of the forehead, and onto the medial pre-frontal cortex at the center of the forehead (where snipers aim). This is why to ensure neuronal-genesis activation, the system of exercise performed must mirror an aggressive act of some sort in order to achieve the "listening behind" response; as, whenever performing Tai Chi. So, this is why, when performing any form in any Tai Chi style, there is usually some set piece of music to accompany the form.

Date: July 8, 2005 10:09:24 PM EDT
Subject: The Thirteen Turns

Regarding your inquiry about the three wheels meditation methodology, and as to what its next level consists of:

1) Imagine a great red circle. Circle is Crimson.

2) Inside this crimson red circle are three wheels spinning.

3) Imagine each wheel as having a different hue, tone, odor.

4) Imagine the three wheels spinning inside the red circle in relationship to each other, as if parts of a machine, and each one is emitting its own distinct hue, tone and odor as it spins; so that there exists a void, an emptiness, in the center about which the three wheels are spinning, and that void is its hub.

5) Now imagine that within each of the three wheels, in their hubs, the empty center of each wheel, another three wheels are spinning, again each one with its own hue, tone and odor.

6) So there are nine wheels spinning, three each within each of the original three wheels, and all spinning in relationship; each wheel is itself emitting its own distinct hue, tone, odor.

7) Each wheel moves: the three great wheels, the nine inner wheels, and crimson red circle also spins; to make thirteen.

The Thirteen Turns.

This is one of the exercises of Crom Cruach and intended to portray an old view of universe, and a true nature of reality.

This is an exercise that's probably pretty ancient and what it does is allow one's psychic abilities to be developed, as it is illustrative of the druidic concept of Reflective Harmony; i.e., that each consciousness, although in itself distinct, contains and reflects all the other consciousnesses, in a harmonious fashion; so that multiple consciousnesses manifest, within a single consciousness, and mutual harmonious manifestation of consciousnesses within consciousness is Cause of Being.

Hope that answers your inquiry. Much more difficult than the three wheels, but it's the next level. There are more levels.

Anyway, that's the next level: The Thirteen Turns.

Bill

BILL O'CONNOR

Poet and Lou's oldest martial arts friend

I met Lou in the '80s, at Leung Shum's Eagle Claw Kung Fu school in New York City—a very traditional Chinese martial arts school. Each class started with handstands against the wall.

Lou and I were trying to do our handstands and cartwheels, but we weren't sixteen. Shum said, "Sometimes this is more for younger people." So we switched to his Wu Tai Chi. Then after a while we felt that we didn't see any of the power we always heard about, such as fajin. I left Shum's school, and Lou stayed.

We went to a few Aaron Banks shows together. Banks [promoter of the Oriental World of Self-Defense events at Madison Square Garden] was still big in New York at that time. He had a big school with various teachers offering different martial arts. He was one of the people who first promoted the Chinese systems.

My martial arts friend Lin Butter was looking for a new teacher when someone told her about Ren. At the time, he had a group of Chinese students in Connecticut. She asked me to accompany her to check out the class. He was the real deal. She gave me Ren's VHS tape on the Chen Tai Chi 38 Form, which I loaned to Lou. After he watched it, Lou said, "Ah, that's what I'm looking for. I'm gonna call the guy up." He made the decision right then.

Lou was always looking for the best. He was attracted to Tai Chi because everybody talks about it as the ultimate. It's like graduating from the more Buddhist Shaolin, then doing postgraduate work in the

KUNG FU generally means the hard work and practice needed to master any art. In this case it is referring to Chinese martial arts. Eagle Claw, or "Ying Jow," is a long-range martial art characterized by precise gripping and twisting of the opponent's limbs.

FAJIN is the explosive power generated from the lower abdomen (dantien).

Taoist systems. It's about transferring energy. It's expanding the scapula. You balloon your body. Here's my body—this isn't it—it's this. The scapula, like wings, open.

There's a whole Tai Chi philosophy. The idea of Tai Chi is that the self disappears. In Tai Chi your self no longer is. So you're overcoming ego. And then gradually there's no more ego. You do Tai Chi and it's gone. That's the ideal. It's part of Taoism. It's not Buddhism, which is very different. In **Taoism** the idea is that the yin and yang come together and then you disappear.

SHAOLIN is a Buddhist temple in China that is the birthplace of both Chan Buddhism and Shaolin martial arts.

TAOISM is a Chinese philosophy focused on finding balance with nature and self. It is central to Tai Chi.

Lou and I would go to Szechuan Garden in Midtown after every class and talk about this stuff. One of the problems before we started Chen Tai Chi was that we were not disappearing. We were not reaching this esoteric goal. We didn't see the power or grow spiritually. We didn't see that it was both the physical and the psychic. We were a little disappointed because we were expecting Nirvana. We weren't there.

Lou was also very interested in the martial arts applications of Tai Chi. But I think Ren thought Lou was not ready for the applications. I may be wrong. But the applications can hurt you. So he may have been just a little careful. For example, he didn't show the full joint locks like I already knew, having grown up with Irish martial arts.

[*Bill demonstrates on Scott.*] Now that's a real wristlock. I'll show you the pressure points. Right here

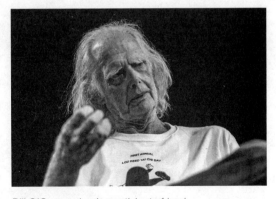

Bill O'Connor, Lou's martial arts friend

is a pressure point, and here is another. What you have to do . . . The trick is to affect the pressure points. You want to connect to pressure points all at once. The training has to do with feeling the points. It's very easy to throw somebody once you control the pressure points, but it takes thousands of hours of practice.

The masters don't immediately tell you the combat application. They tell you the poem for the application. It's a code. So if you don't under- stand Chinese or don't have knowledge of these codes, it's hard to learn. For every form there is a poem that if you memorize, you retain the form.

In the later years, Lou and I mostly talked about Taoism and Buddhism. I always had a problem with those philosophies, because I thought they were missing the point. It's about nothingness. To be a creative there has to be nothingness, because everything else is an assumption when you think it's divided like yin and yang. Maybe you already made a mistake when you think the world is divided into yin and yang. It's not divided. Nothing is more than a whole, like a black hole, which is nothingness. But there's energy spewing out of it. That's what it's about.

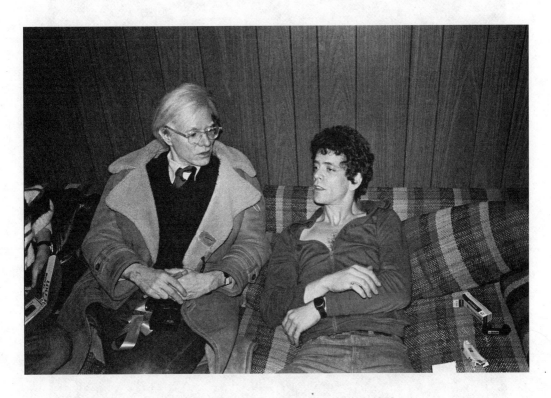

Lou with his friend and mentor Andy Warhol, 1976

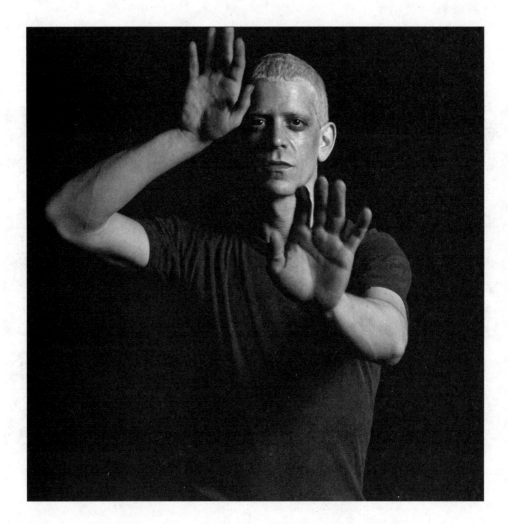

From a photo shoot by Mick Rock, 1974

CHAPTER 2

STARTING OUT

Doin' the things that we want to

My first Tai Chi teacher, Leung Shum, studied from the age of six. My current teacher, Ren GuangYi, studied Tai Chi since he was seventeen. His teacher, Chen Xiaowang, has a son, Chen Pengfei, who won his first tournament at three!

—FROM "LOU REED: THE TAIJI RAVEN SPEAKS,"
BY MARTHA BURR, *KUNG FU TAI CHI* MAGAZINE, MAY/JUNE 2003

From an interview with Lou for Rock On, BBC Radio 1, March 26, 1983, presenter Richard Skinner, producer Pete Ritzema

BBC: You're looking in better health than I've ever seen you.

LOU REED: Oh, well, thanks. I do appreciate that.

BBC: Is that the reason you've been consciously working out?

LOU: Yeah, I've been consciously getting in good shape. I suppose you want to know how? I worked out, and one of the nice things that happened to me is my wife Sylvia's brother, Peter, is a Kung Fu weapons tournament champ—which he has been for a very long time. And he's gone through a number of different systems, mainly starting with Kenpo, ending up with Long Fist Kung Fu, and I studied with Peter for a long time.

BBC: What's the name of the system that you use?

LOU: Wu-style Tai Chi Chuan, Chinese boxing.

BBC: Has taking part in the classes made you

KENPO is a modern martial art based on Chinese martial arts and Karate. Long Fist, or "Chang Chuan," is a long-range martial art from northern China that relies on extended arm and leg strikes to keep the opponent at a distance.

much more aware about looking after your body? And the importance of eating the right things?

LOU: And learning the meaning of the word "pain." [*Laughs awkwardly*.] That particular kind of training is useful in working off tension the way a motorcycle does for me—same thing.

MERRILL WEINER

Lou's sister

Our grandfather's name was Mendel Rabinowitz. You may notice that it is Jewish. Our father worked for the unions at a time when unions were considered Communist. He changed the family name to Reed for protection. I don't know if that was really it or if it was our Jewish identity. They had a son, Lewis Allan Reed, and then me, Margaret Ellen Reed. I changed my name to Merrill when I graduated college. I always thought they should have just named me Madonna and admitted their trouble with Judaism. I think our father deprived us of having beliefs, and Lou was very spiritual. We didn't really celebrate holidays. There was no big Christmas. There was no Hanukkah. Passover was just family over for dinner. That's the claustrophobic place I think Lou had to break out of. Home was intolerable for him. Our cousin Shirley was the Commie, the Norma Rae of the garment workers. They were close. She really became his spiritual mother in many, many ways.

Lou wasn't a teasing older brother—maybe the opposite. Once when he was babysitting me there was a spider in my room. He wouldn't go in. He refused to kill it. I was incensed. Many years later I was going to school in Cleveland and the Velvet Underground came to play. It would have been about 1966. I went to see them, and Lou said, "Bunny, don't tell anyone we're related." I assume he just wanted people to think he sprang out of the earth like a flower, but still I was the younger sister and I adored him. I would forgive him for anything.

"Hello, Bunny. It's Lou." It's that sound. That voice, not the singing voice, the speaking one. It was beautiful—it was like music. He is present in my mind so much of the time.

Both of us loved the martial arts. For a birthday he gave me the entire catalog of Bruce Lee. My understanding is his real introduction to martial arts came from his second wife, Sylvia. He met her brother, who was a successful martial artist and taught Lou. Over time, I feel Lou's passion for Tai Chi became more spiritual. He became a better version of himself and became an elder statesman. As he developed, even more so with Ren, he understood the discipline in a profound way, and it brought him some peace of mind.

His vision was so large, and he was relentless. Nothing stopped him. That is what made him. He was also a genius. That vision encompassed Tai Chi and music, as well as simpler things like designing the perfect roller bag or a new kind of eyeglasses.

When my husband and I got married, Lou had been in the Velvet Underground, but now he was living at home. I remember Harold saying, "I hope you don't have to support your brother."

JONATHAN RICHMAN

Velvet Underground fan, musician, songwriter, stonemason

I, as a sixteen-year-old, was actually an upset high school student. I was walking around Harvard Square a few days before a Velvet Underground show at the Boston Tea Party, and a guy with a guitar case was walking through on that beautiful spring afternoon. And I said, "Excuse me. Are you Lou Reed?" And he says, "Yes." I told him that his music meant so much to me, and he said, "Can I ask what you like about it?" And I said, "For one thing, you use the guitars as percussion instruments." He says, "Really? You get that from it?" I said yes. And he said, "You mean use them as drums?" I said, "Yeah. In certain songs, yeah."

I guess he liked what I said, so I was in. They let me see the Velvet Underground but also let me not just watch as someone from the seats, but they let me show up early while the group was bringing in their stuff. And they were all nice to me. Sterling Morrison and John Cale, they were all sitting around. From this point on, this group . . . My gratitude cannot be really expressed in words. I get misty when I try and talk about it. They would just let me study them. Lou Reed, after a while, would let me try out his electric guitars during their rehearsals and just listen to the sounds.

I would say, "How come you use the midrange boost, and the fuzz tone like that at the same time?" And Lou would say, "Well, this gives you this." And he would show me! This group that was so known for being foreboding, even among themselves, were so nice to me.

I met Andy Warhol at the same time. He could be standoffish if he wanted to. He asked me about high school. And I said, "Well, I don't feel very well understood there, and I get scared by it sometimes." And he said, "Uh-huh." It didn't seem alien to him. "Look, when you graduate high school, come down to New York and you can work with me on films." He was big on education and hard work. Within a few months, he got shot. I went down and he remembered who I was. He was the same but not the same. He couldn't have the hands-on thing in his movies anymore, but there I was in New York, near them, and near that scene and the Velvet Underground.

I had seen the Velvet Underground between sixty and a hundred times. And my parents, bless their hearts, let me go see these weirdos.

And I explained who they were, and they knew who Andy Warhol was, but they trusted me. And they were right to, because I actually was what I said I was. As a painter, I heard their sound. And it wasn't just the lyrics, although Lou Reed gave me my voice as a singer.

But their sound, their actual sound of the drones and their atmospheres. I was just learning to do bar chords and things like that. Sterling Morrison and Lou Reed taught me how to play. Sterling would say, "Jonathan, do you know how to do this chord?" I said, "No. Which is that?" "This is another way to do a C chord. Can you get your finger to bend like that?" And I'd say, "Yeah, I guess I can." "Okay, you already know this stuff, the Chuck Berry stuff, right?" I'd say, "No. I don't know any of this stuff." Sterling Morrison especially taught me how to play guitar. I would say, "Lou, can you tell me why you use this tone

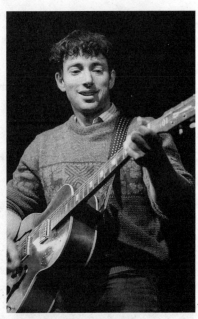

Jonathan Richman in performance, 1986

rather than that one. . . . How did you get that?" And then Lou Reed would say, "Ah, young man, that was many things." They would make fun of me as a mascot, but I wasn't concerned. I knew I deserved it, but also, mainly, they were letting me learn. I almost didn't care what they said. And if you don't think I'm grateful, I'm almost tripping right now. I can barely say it. I was sixteen and it was life or death for me.

Lou Reed was one of the people who got me on a spiritual path. Mitch Blake was the custodian of the Boston Tea Party club, and he became an older-brother figure to me. They brought me to the local natural-food restaurant called Erewhon, one of the first macrobiotic restaurants in New England.

Maureen Tucker was great with me. John Cale was standoffish but was also great and would talk to me sometimes. He didn't talk much period, but they would let me in their dressing room. When their dressing room was there in the back of the Boston Tea Party, I was there! They would let me listen to band arguments about tuning, about stuff like this! Even then I realized the oddness of this. I was saying, "They're letting me hang around for this?"

And, I would watch their hands. I would watch them play guitar during rehearsal. I'd watch them onstage. I learned how to improvise from them. I would watch them make up songs. . . . They would use their sound checks, and sound checks back then were a primitive affair for everyone. There was almost no such thing as monitor speakers. There was none of the loud sound checks that have become what a modern sound check

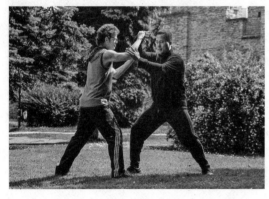

Training on tour in Europe, mid-2000s

is. In 1968, a sound check was, a band would more or less make sure everything worked. But they would stay onstage enough hours, they would just work out new material. "I Heard Her Call My Name," "Beginning to See the Light," "I'm Set Free," "Jesus" . . . I heard them work out all these songs, and Lou Reed would put down one guitar and pick up a Fender twelve-string for another. He'd let me play that Fender twelve-string or something.

Around that time, I actually opened up for them at a place around Boston called the Woodrose Ballroom. After that, for no apparent reason, Lou cut me off. I offended him in some way that I didn't know. Sterling Morrison would just say, "Oh, he's like that." I remember once it happened, he didn't speak to me for years. And I got over it, and I just figured,

Okay. If I'm on my own, the heavens must want me to be on my own and take my own path. Lou and I would talk mystical stuff occasionally, and he would tell me about mystical books and things. I'd say, *I wonder if he's cutting me off for two reasons. One, because I'm obnoxious, and maybe also he might be trying to do me some favor.* I'll never know the answer.

So Lou was into meditation by that point. He in fact would go to these monthly meditations that the Alice Bailey people had at the United Nations. Lou Reed would tell me about the Alice Bailey Lucis Trust books. People who go to mystic bookstores will be familiar with books like *A Treatise on White Magic* and *A Treatise on Cosmic Fire*. He would talk to me about stuff like this. It's also in some of his songs. Like "Over the hill we go, and you're looking for love," the words like "Insects are evil thoughts"—this is from that material. The idea of manifestations of certain thoughts being physically sometimes, in the animal kingdom, positive or negative. Lou was into stuff like that, and he told me, "When you move to New York, go to the moon meditations at the United Nations. I go there sometimes."

The next time I spoke with him was in 1992. So all the time that he was Lou Reed the solo performer, I had musician friends who knew him. And actually, they were on instructions. They would say, "Oh, we're friends of Jonathan," and he would say, "Don't give him my phone number."

In 1992, I had a show in New York at the Lone Star Roadhouse, and Penn Jillette invited Lou to come to the show. After the show, Penn and Teller took about eight of us to a Midtown deli. Lou sat next to me and said, "You know, Jonathan, having seen you play tonight, I'm proud of you." And I was sixteen again. I was already about thirty-eight or forty years old at that time. And he said, "And I know what that means to you."

You should know, in addition to music, my other job is that I build bread ovens. I've still got to be outside, doing things, and I was like that all my life. I'm a stonemason. I've also studied a bit of martial arts and in San Francisco found a school of Tai Chi in the Cheng Man-ch'ing tradition. My favorite thing about Tai Chi is the philosophy of it. It makes me laugh, because it's so non-macho, and it shows how non-macho works over macho. If you've been in a Push Hands class with a heavier person pushing against you, as long as your arms are soft enough and you don't resist, he will just topple himself.

In a Tai Chi magazine, I read Push Hands described as an exercise in temperament. It took me five years to let people push me around. Finally, though, I did. Finally, I got to the point where . . . Because the instructor said to me, "Jonathan, we expect you, as someone who's been here awhile, you follow the rules in Push Hands. If a beginner doesn't or if an advanced student doesn't, that's their problem. You don't reprimand them; you don't do shit. You just stick with the rules and let them push you over, and that's the end of it."

Apparently, Lou had a poem, "Seventeen-year-old Jonathan asks me if he should take drugs, and I tell him no." And I thought, *Thank God*, because I would've made the worst drug addict you ever saw, because I was terrified of needles, and also, I was always active. I would say, "Lou, do I need these drugs?" He'd say, "No, Jonathan, you don't." That's the Lou Reed I knew, incidentally: introspective, eager to share insight, curious, open to new ideas—musically and spiritually. People emphasize the drug aspect in his music. Well, what I got from it had nothing to do with any of that. What I got from it was much more a spiritual vibe from the music of the band as a whole.

One of the first things we were taught is, any state you could achieve with chemicals, you could achieve with silence. I like to move slowly, which incidentally helps my meditation. An oxcart pace, as someone put it. I'm not much of a participant in the computer age.

SYLVIA REED

Lou's second wife, manager, designer, and collaborator in the 1980s

I met Lou at a time when he was deeply impacted by years of heavy drug and alcohol abuse that were detrimental to his health and work. He was struggling to find his way out of an intense cycle of self-destruction. I provided a catalyst that he welcomed to initiate a change in his life. He knew that his life was in danger if he could not stop the use of substances. So when we married in 1980, he made a commitment to change these patterns. One part of his new ambition to regain his health involved the martial arts.

I believe that Lou had first been made aware of martial arts by one of the musicians who worked with him who may have had some experience. As we spent more time together, I was able to provide him with more in-depth information, based on my own experience training in the arts as a teenager, learning from my brother.

My older brother Peter was already studying the martial arts in his high school years, when we lived in Taiwan and in Hawaii. Peter was Lou's first martial arts teacher.

We often went to a theater in Chinatown to see Kung Fu movies which were always being screened. He also loved to watch Bruce Lee movies and we'd talk about the power of his form. Lou grasped this part of the art right away, and he learned to recognize which martial artist was performing at the highest level when we watched tournaments. In the couple of years Peter was working with him, he was struck with just how serious the martial arts became to Lou. It was not a passing fancy. His martial arts practice would become an important part of his life over the years. My brother's time as Lou's teacher came to an end in the mid-1980s, when Peter enrolled in law school and pursued a legal career.

Lou and I had noticed a martial arts studio in New York, on the second floor of a building at Ninth Avenue and 34th Street. This was the studio of Master Leung Shum. Finally, one day we decided to enter the studio and take a look at the classes. We began taking private lessons to learn the long form Tai Chi with Master Shum. Master Shum was generous with his time, but not his praise. He expected a student to work hard to improve.

It's notable that this practice was not something that came naturally to Lou. It was different with his songwriting, which came so easily to him that many people have witnessed his ability to play something on the guitar and almost instantly come up with strong lyrics that no one else could write. To learn these martial arts forms demanded all his focus and it took him months to make the movements of even part of one form come together. It demanded a lot of his energy as well, and there were times when he felt exhausted and discouraged that he wasn't moving smoothly or that he was forgetting sections of a form. He used handwritten notes to remind himself of the particular choreography. He painstakingly wrote out "Step with left foot while pushing with right arm and lifting," "lean backward with shoulders steady and twist right foot." I think just the act of writing it down allowed him to access the information in a way that helped him, until it could become part of muscle memory. Later, Lou began studying with Master Larry Tan.

Having heard from quite a few people that Lou practiced with in his later years, I'm very glad to know that he came to a place where he could actually teach someone else. I think that has a lot of significance. Lou had a gracious and generous side to him that not many people were aware of. I remember him being open and kind when a friend was in need. But patience never came naturally to him. I think patience is another gift that martial arts gave to him. People he knew in his classes have described how he helped them with a gentle "Okay, this is how you do it." What people often don't realize about him is that he was really collaborative. He enjoyed building a song with musicians, pulling a show together with other creative people. But in the musical world he was always the center of the project. To be a teacher in an area where he was not the focus is a very different thing, and I was happy to know that he developed the ability to open up and share like that.

This renewed strength and health did lead to a professional transition. He was at such a point before becoming sober that people in the business weren't sure if he would make it through a show or if he would show up for the next tour. But in subsequent years he became an artist who was lauded for his productivity, reliability, and commitment. I think it was his martial arts practice that was a great resource for him during this time. During these years of intense work, I do remember him as being happy, creatively engaged, and that he found great joy in his life. Lou found strength in both his music and in the martial arts and it was these two lifelong interests that allowed him to share his gifts with us.

MICK ROCK

Photographer who shot many iconic images of Lou

Lou pushed the limits quite a lot. I remember after four days with no sleep I kind of said, "I think the time has come," and he said to me, "Mick, don't be a pussy. We're only just beginning." And he carried on longer. I mean he did push the envelope more than most people I knew. But he was

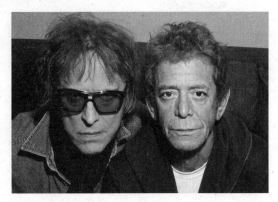

Mick and Lou at a book signing, 2013

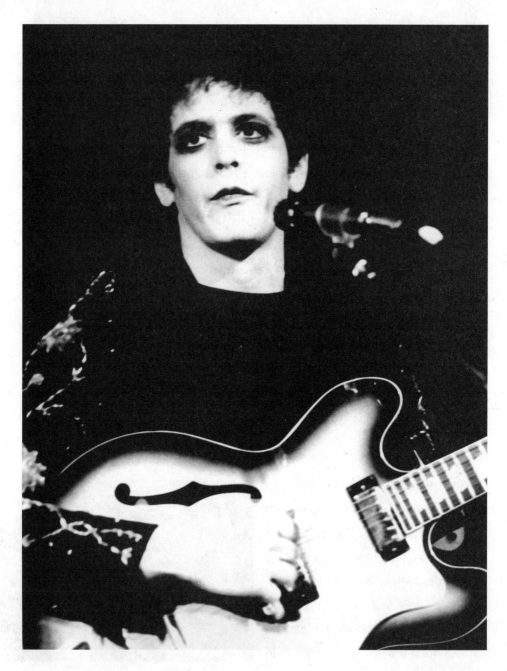

Cover of Transformer, photo by Mick Rock, 1976

always exploring different things. His energy came from a number of things. One is his infinite curiosity, and of course there was a little help from the stimulants. He always had a book on something, and he always had a new tape recorder, and he was always taking me to a Barnes & Noble and showing me some very esoteric books. His intellectual capacity was huge.

He would show me scientific books that would explain certain things, including exploring stimulants and what they did to him, and he wasn't just someone who would do something. He wanted to know what it was doing to his system. I think it was inevitable that Lou would get into some discipline, like the martial arts, because I think he'd gotten to the end of where stimulants could take him, and he wasn't going to be victimized by it, ultimately. We spent a lot of time together; it was a different time. Those long nights or days. I started doing the Hatha Yoga very early on. He thought it was interesting that I was into it, but he wasn't quite ready to jump into one of those disciplines. There may be somewhere pictures of me doing headstands. I remember him writing about me doing headstands at some point, and cocaine. I think he really liked the irony of that.

SHARYN FELDER

Friend, daughter of the songwriter Doc Pomus, Lou's mentor

Lou told me that the way he met my father was he looked him up in the phone book. He was listed. Lou called Dad out of the blue and they just became friends. This was in the early '80s. My dad was giving a workshop. It was really fifteen students mostly in their twenties. Maybe seven classes, like a master class. They'd each write a song and come back and everybody would hear it. Lou came and listened to the songs. He was very respectful and he commented on them. Legendary song-writers came like Otis Blackwell from the Brill Building, Jerry Leiber or Mike Stoller, Tom Waits; they all came but I was very intimidated by Lou because I idolized him.

Lou was really eager to hear all of the ins and outs of the business. He was really struggling with stuff. He was very unhappy with the record companies, with managers. My dad was giving him wisdom. Lou said later that my father always said "Consider the source, Lou."

My father was a large guy in a wheelchair, songwriter, originally a singer. His songwriting was very direct and he really liked to give a lot. He nurtured people. I think he really looked to Lou to try to help him.

Straight arrow kind of thing and that's how he was as a person. Lou always said that to me, "He's like a straight shooter, no bullshit." His song-writing was kind of like that. The shortest distance, the straight line thing in the words. Irving Berlin was his songwriting mentor.

It's just using the word always, repeating it. I was thinking, lines like Lou said once to me, he wished my father broke out of that chorus verse line. Because that was the old school. Lou liked a very direct approach. "Just do it. Don't second-guess" was always his advice.

My father worked fast. We have footage of him writing the lyrics. He liked to write that way, writing on a napkin, on a matchbook. My mother said their early marriage, all the songs are inside of paperback books.

That is so pure. My dad was a very pure person. Even in the journals he wrote. It's funny, I saw something in Lou's writing, "I always believed in magic, and flying." That was an opening line of one of my dad's journal entries. That was in the 1940s.

LAURIE ANDERSON: You're kidding? It was *Magic and Loss*.

SHARYN FELDER: *Magic and Loss*, exactly. They both had something about flying. They both came from Brooklyn, twenty years apart. My dad came from Williamsburg. Both of them came from families that didn't understand them exactly.

My dad's parents were obsessed with how their son was going to make it in the world. They envisioned him as somebody who would be selling pencils in the street. They would bring, like, the insurance salesman to the house, "Could you learn this trade?"

I found a letter maybe only four, five years ago from FDR to my grandmother. He was governor of New York saying, "Dear Mrs. Felder. I'm so sorry about your little boy." I don't know how I never found that letter before.

My dad was a real outsider because of his disability. He always connected to outsiders. Not just the crazy Jewish outsiders. Because around then all of his girlfriends were Black. He always identified Black when he was a kid. He got polio when he was six.

He started as a blues singer, a white guy on crutches in an all-Black band.

Lou and Dad had some kind of a deep connection. Between the late '80s and '91, Lou was on the phone with him all the time, coming by, calling for advice. My dad would always say, "Just got off the phone with Lou. We had a really nice talk."

When my dad was diagnosed with lung cancer, it was very aggressive, very fast. You go into the hospital and you just don't come out.

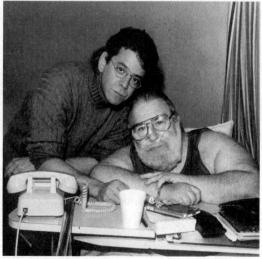

Lou visiting Doc Pomus in the hospital

When he got sick Lou started coming to the hospital every day, which was really intense. Lou would say to me things like, "He can't go. He's like the sun." That's what he kept saying, "He's like the sun." I think he was writing the album already.

He was in for a month before he died. A month, maybe two, between diagnosis and death. That was '91. Lou came every day. It was like he was going to work. We saw a lot of him in the hospital. He brought the song "What's Good" in to my dad and my dad listened to that in the hospital. I don't think he could quite wrap his head around the concept—he was dying but he would say, "Can you believe it? Lou wrote a song for me."

I kept thinking, *I don't know him that well to be there all the time with him.* I felt it was something that was helping him too, like it was a healing thing for him. I just felt that he needed to be there.

He died March 14 of '91. *Magic and Loss* came out January 1992. I asked Lou to speak at the funeral. He was really great.

He said, "Doc said that he would like to go to Katz's Deli with me to have a Knoblewurst. Which is kind of a hot dog, a more serious kind of hot dog. Like a real bratwurst, but super Jewy, Knoblewurst. Then he ended with 'I'll save the last dance for him or he'll save the last dance for me. . . .'" Something like that. Everybody was crying. Lou took it very, very seriously.

I remember years later when he came to my house. I was making a documentary and Jimmy Scott was there and Lou said to Jimmy, "Could you be my teacher?" Jimmy said, "Yeah baby."

Jimmy taught him to sing vibrato. He said, "It's easy Lou, you just sing one note and then sing a little below it. Then keep that up until the notes get closer." Like that, that's vibrato. Then he started using vibrato in all his stuff.

We made a tribute album to my dad in '92. Lou picked "This Magic Moment" to play. He couldn't believe it when I told him that song was available and he was the best person to do it.

My dad was a boxing fanatic. When he died, I gave Lou a lot of his boxing tapes. He liked martial arts, he liked weapons too. He had swords. He had all kinds of weapons. He never used them but he and Lou shared the love of boxing and the martial arts.

It's funny, I'm thinking about some of the titles that he wrote years before he knew Lou. "Power and the Glory" is also a name of a song he wrote. He liked larger-than-life things. He saw himself as somebody that was larger than life, never as a disabled person. I think he connected to Lou in some of this muscularity kind of thing.

He lived alone towards the end of his life and he was in bed. Once you would help him get into bed, he needed another person to help him out. He had a button on the side of the bed to open the front door. Because he would order food and have deliveries and stuff. He kept a gun in the bed.

Later when Lou and I were neighbors in Springs on Long Island I think he compartmentalized me a little bit in the sense that he always wanted to talk about music. A lot of it was music. He really was a musicologist. He knew a lot of obscure information—just the details of stuff. We talked about beauty, the light. I took him to different beaches he'd never been to. I showed him around.

He tried to teach me Tai Chi too. He told me that my trunk was very strong. I thought, *Yes! I could do this*. He said you are as old as your legs. It made me feel, like, very powerful.

Lou wanted to learn, he was that way. Every time I saw him with Ralph Gibson or whomever, it was like once he had a way of seeing you, then that's how he always saw you. Like every time I saw him with Ralph, he wanted to get into something with him, learn more about the camera. He was very fixated on learning.

Even his anger was beautiful because there was always a truth in it. He would always quote my dad. "Consider the source." I can picture him doing these little gesture things. In his later years he would always say, "Aren't we lucky?" He said that to me so many times, "Aren't we lucky?" Meaning that we were out in Springs. That was something he said a lot. He loved watching my dog Betty running and said, "I wish I was a dog."

PETER MORALES

American pioneer and champion of Chinese-style martial arts, Lou's first teacher

My sister Sylvia told me she was seeing this gentleman named Lou Reed. I had no idea who he was. I'd never heard a lick of his music. I stopped in New York on my way to Germany and she told me all about him. There was no mention of martial arts. I mean she always knew I was into martial arts then, but we didn't talk about that.

When I met Lou, Sylvia told me that he was trying to get off drugs, including heroin. I remember seeing the tracks on his arms. I saw an individual who physically was capable of doing martial arts, who was strong. But it looked like he had abused his body. I saw a strong person who was in a state of spiritual fatigue. We're talking about 1978 when I met him. But at that time, the notion of me teaching him did not come up. Before they got married, Sylvia said she was looking for a way to help Lou get his body straightened out. She told me he was struggling with heroin use.

She said that the reason she wanted to introduce him to me was because I was a complete martial arts obsessive. She said, "He's kind of an obsessive, and if he gets obsessed with the martial arts, what harm can it do?"

But I didn't know what he was going through. Sometimes at dinner, after a training session, he would talk about some of the things he'd been going through. It became clear to me that a life in music, even when you're successful, is an incredibly difficult life. I was happy that he was open to a system that I thought could be of some help physically and spiritually. And Sylvia was right that he was an obsessive.

It began as a series of cross-country flights. I would fly into Newark and be driven to their Blairstown, New Jersey, home for weekend—if not longer—training. I remember being in Blairstown at least once per month for quite a while. And that's where all of the training would take place. It was completely isolated. We would train by a beautiful pond almost like in Kung Fu movies!

He was given an intensive course in the martial arts. We would do a session, for an hour or two. He was being fed a lot, much more than any other

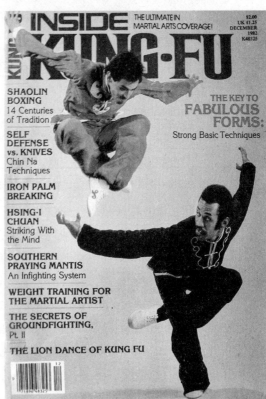

Lou's first martial arts teacher Peter Morales (in the air) on the cover of Inside Kung Fu *magazine (with Dennis Brown), December 1982*

student would get, because we knew that I was only there for three days. We'd have a morning session. Then lunch, followed by walking and talking around the pond, or he'd go off to work on his music. After lunch, we'd have an afternoon session and sometimes even an evening session. At the very least, it was twice per day, if not three times.

I started training him specifically on three or four different things, but none of them were Tai Chi. I trained him in Chuan Fa. He had a very interesting reaction to all of it. He was like a kid in a candy store. He had no idea how expansive the martial arts were. There were a few moments when he was very fascinated by the movement but didn't realize that they were all fighting movements. And when he asked me what it meant, I still remember the surprise in his eyes when I said, "Let me show you what Praying Mantis is about." He even asked me to teach him and his bodyguard a few times.

CHUAN FA: Before 1949, Chinese martial arts, including Eagle Claw and Praying Mantis, were referred to as Chuan Fa, or "Fist Method."

The crucial moment came when he finally asked, "Well, what does this stuff do?" I said, "You don't understand. These are all self-defense gestures, based on the movements of animals." He had a love-at-first-sight moment when he realized these movements came from the genius of ancient Chinese people who studied animals, which we often see in martial arts movies.

Lou came at it from an intellectual sense, unlike many other people. Most of them are, "I want to know what it does," which is not unusual. There's nothing wrong with that, because I think any good teacher is going to have somebody eventually ask, "Well, how do you use this?" With Lou, because we weren't seeing each other as often as the usual student-teacher situation, I wanted to keep him fascinated, because we were trying to help him understand his body and get on his road to a good sense of health. After one occasion when I showed him the meaning of a movement, it was, for me, that moment as an instructor when you realize, *Okay, this guy gets it. He's fascinated with it. I'm not going to have any more selling to do. I just have to teach him now.*

He was always attentive and raring to go. After a while, his needle tracks weren't there anymore, as he became more fascinated with the arts and seemed more reliant on them.

WUSHU, or "war arts," is the term that came into wide use on mainland China after 1949 as the generic term for Chinese martial arts.

There was a martial arts revolution going on at that time in the US. And Wushu was at the forefront of that. Lou was part of that martial arts wave going on in the '80s. One event I remember was in Chicago. He got to see one of the best Wushu players in the world, Anthony Chan, perform Chang Chuan. Lou was floored by it. I remember this because I was surprised that he was willing to come to the tournament, because he was there for a concert.

I remember reading about his having Ren perform onstage with him. I was happy about that. I thought that was a tribute. I thought that was just his being very proud of a part of his life and revealing it to other people in a way that he probably wouldn't reveal other parts of his life.

He was always fascinated by the history. He was fascinated by these odd stories of someone studying the movements of the Praying Mantis and being able to turn it into a human self-defense system.

For a long time, he kept it to himself. I think he liked keeping it a bit of a secret from people, at least while he was learning. I think it's surprising to many people when they think about Lou Reed—they know about the persona that created such great music but do not know that he was grounded by the martial arts.

I introduced him to Leung Shum's school. I took him to a class so he could see the studio. I last saw him on Christopher Street in the '90s.

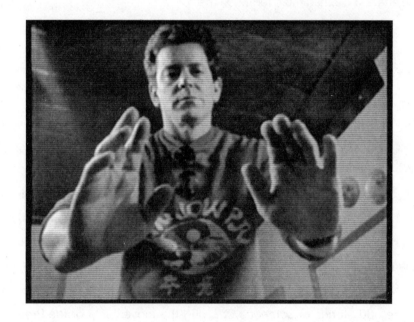

Lou in the Jim Carroll video for "Sweet Jane," 1983

It was clear that he felt comfortable enough to speak with some authority about various principles. He had come into his own with it. I watched the transformation of a person who literally ran into something he knew nothing about, but the more he learned martial arts, the more quiet and respectful of the arts he became.

EDITOR'S NOTE: SCOTT RICHMAN

During research for this book, I visited the Lou Reed Archive at the New York Public Library, spending several hours listening to un-released audio, including rough mixes, demos, and alternate ver-sions of Lou's solo and Velvet Underground material. In a digital file labeled "Demos and Rehearsals Lou Reed Outs #560558," I lis-tened to an unlabeled song and as it played through, the lyrics were unfamiliar and were describing his experience with Tai Chi Chuan, talking about his first martial arts teacher, Peter Morales. The unre-leased song, that we titled "Open Invitation," was recorded during the sessions for 1986's *Mistrial* recorded at the Power Station in New York City. A sample of the lyrics include:

An open invitation, to Tai Chi Chuan
An open invitation, to Tai Chi Chuan

The last time I saw Peter, he went to The Orient
He was doing a little Wushu, and he showed me some of it
He did the Praying Mantis and he taught a form to me
And then over dinner, he showed me some Tai Chi

LEUNG SHUM

Eagle Claw Kung Fu grandmaster and Lou's second martial arts teacher and first Tai Chi instructor

Lou first came to me in the early 1980s. He said, "Sifu, I really want to learn Tai Chi, but I can't find a good teacher. I don't want a group class, because I can't learn easily. So can you teach me privately?"

When he first started, it was not easy for me. Because he was very shaky when he moved his hands. It was very hard for him to learn just

SIFU in Cantonese Chinese, or "shih fu" in Mandarin Chinese, is an honorific meaning father-teacher.

a few movements. I asked, "Why are you shaking?" I tried very hard. After a few one-hour sessions, he only learned six movements, but not very well. I said, "How about next time you come, I don't want you shaking. When you're shaking I can't teach you. You try. Don't shake. Try to slow down by yourself. Go slowly." And then he said, "Okay. I'll try. I'll practice at home, these few movements."

The next day, I said, "I can't teach you, because it is very hard for me to teach you. I spend one hour to only teach you a few movements. But Tai Chi forms have hundreds of movements." I told him it takes a long time to learn. He insisted, "Sifu, I beg you. Please, please. Really. I really want to learn it."

After only a few weeks, he did not improve. I yelled at him. "If you want to learn good Tai Chi, you should stop doing drugs and drinking! I don't want to teach you." So after that, he got a little angry and left. But after two weeks, he returned and said, "Sifu, I'm sorry. I really want to learn this. Can you teach me again? Please,

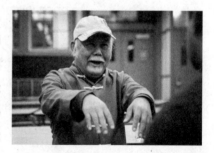

Master Leung Shum demonstrating Tai Chi

please, please?" I say, "Yeah, you really want it? Why do you want this?" He said, "Because I want to be stronger."

I said, "Okay. If you want to learn it, I'll continue to try. But don't say I wasted your time. If you're no good, I can't teach you. It's up to you to get it." The next time he came feeling better. He said, "Okay, today is better. I'll try." He was much better. I taught him some more. After those classes, he learned quicker. He continued slowly for about four years.

He was smart and also hardworking. He told me, "Sifu, I practice at home every day." I said, "Very nice, good." He got better and better—with no more shaking. I said to him, "Your body was really weak up to now, but you're beginning to get strong and better." His stepping got better, and he finished the first form very nicely. He then learned the second form very well.

Lou's notes from his Tai Chi practice, mid-'80s

Then he said to me, "Sifu, I want to learn fighting!" I said, "Lou, you fighting is not good, because your body is still weak. Try to get stronger. First make the form better. Learning how to fight is not going to happen. First make your body stronger. Keep practicing, your body will be naturally strong. When you're strong, you can do everything you want."

I told him, "Why are you in such a hurry? You're still young." And then later I said, "If you want to fight, I'll teach you the basics of fighting—how to protect yourself first." He learned these basics very well. He also learned Tui Shou [Push Hands].

He asked me, "Sifu, can I write a Tai Chi song?" I said, "Yeah, very good." He specially made it and put it on cassette. The song was missing important things about Tai Chi—a lot of the internal things. He just sang about making a circle. That's it. Nothing else. He didn't sing about what's inside Tai Chi.

LAURIE ANDERSON: Lou talked about Eagle Claw as a guitar player. He said that really changed him and made it possible to use his hands differently. Did he talk to you about that?

LEUNG SHUM: Eagle Claw can train your fingers to be strong and very smooth. So maybe it can help improve guitar playing. Lou told me he had diabetes. I have diabetes too. My diabetes is serious. But why am I still strong? Because of Tai Chi—I can say that. It makes me strong! People say that if you keep doing Tai Chi, you'll always improve and never get old.

LAURIE: Tai Chi, you'll always improve and never get old. You have to first get stronger internally.

LEUNG: You have to first get stronger internally. Tai Chi is the best way to keep you alive and to keep you strong. It makes the internal organs strong. You get better and better. How can you get sick again?

LARRY TAN

Lou's third martial arts teacher, who trained him in self-defense

Lou and I met in '83 at Leung Shum's school. A student there introduced me to Lou. Billy Idol was my student at that time, so Lou was curious.

Shum is a great master of Eagle Claw and also a Tai Chi master. Lou focused more on Tai Chi. And when we started talking, Lou was very interested in both the health and combat aspects. I explained to him that because Shum is teaching Tai Chi in a very traditional manner, if he wanted to learn practical self-defense, it would take a long time. I said, "Look at Bruce Lee," and Lou was an avid fan of Lee. I said, this is what Bruce Lee was teaching, who was updating martial arts. But because I'm also traditional in many ways, I appreciate that you have to go back to the roots to understand what they were really teaching thousands of years ago.

Lou started coming to me weekly for private training. We kept his training with me quiet, because he was a student of Shum and wanted to show respect. I would take the bus to his home in New Jersey. He'd pick me up on his Harley! He loved Tai Chi. He loved martial arts. . . . There were a few times we watched the famous Hagler–Leonard boxing fight together. He loved boxing matches!

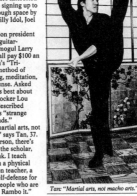

THE HANDS OF TAN

IN A TRANQUIL UPPER EAST SIDE STUDIO, real-estate developer Marc DiLorenzo is balancing on one leg. With a shout, he thrusts out with a vicious side kick. "No," says a slim Asian-American man. "Look." And with a small, almost gentle flick, kung fu master Larry Tan sends DiLorenzo flying across the room. "*Align* your body," says Tan. "*Feel* your balance."

Helping DiLorenzo up, he gives a little smile. "Power," he says with a nod. "It's really just proper alignment."

New Yorkers interested in power are signing up to be flung through space by Larry Tan. Billy Idol, Joel Grey, Carey Transportation president Peter Price, guitar-electronics mogul Larry DiMarzio—all pay $100 an hour for Tan's "Tri-Harmony" method of bodybuilding, meditation, and self-defense. Asked what he likes best about New York, rocker Lou Reed once described Master Tan's "strange dazzling hands."

"I teach martial arts, not macho arts," says Tan, 37. "In every person, there's the warrior, the scholar, and the monk. I teach them all. I'm a physical trainer, a Zen teacher, a therapist. Self-defense for intelligent people who are not going to Rambo it."

Tan grew up a Queens street kid, but his grandfather, Tsou Lu, was among the founding fathers of modern China—he fought with Sun Yat-sen. After college, Tan traveled through Asia for seven years, learning about his past, honing his craft—and starring in kung fu movies. He returned to America and became a martial-arts coordinator for such films as *The Wanderers* and *The Exterminator*. Seven years ago, he began teaching, turning students into fierce advocates.

"I can apply what Tan shows me directly to business," says Larry DiMarzio. "Know your opponent, know yourself. Learn when to go toe-to-toe, when to wait and jump them from a tree."

Lou Reed applies the training in another way. While he was in the studio working on his latest album, *Mistrial*, the atmosphere became tense, explosive. Reed went into another room and practiced Tan's "Universal Form" until he was calm.

"You can only do so many reps on the Nautilus machine," says Marc DiLorenzo. "But with kung fu, there's a whole history, a whole grace, a whole knowledge. It's so much more than just pushing a dumbbell."

ROBERT GOLDBERG

Tan: "Martial arts, not macho arts."

Lou's third martial arts teacher, Larry Tan, featured in New York magazine, 1986

He was so passionate about martial arts, and he was really curious about my trying to teach martial arts as practical self-defense and how to accelerate that process. I was trying to be the bridge between traditional martial arts, which he was studying and didn't fully understand then, and modern combat. I'm the guy who taught Lou how to fight.

There were some breaks in his training, and when we got back together, we'd focus. I taught him a system that I was creating at the time. I was a martial art rebel who was trying to understand traditional Chinese martial arts but was also heavily influenced by Bruce Lee, who was trying to modernize martial arts. My whole life had been trying to bridge modern martial arts with the traditional arts. Lou was very sweet. He mentioned me in *New York* magazine and also in an interview for a martial arts magazine. Fernando Saunders also began studying with me from an introduction by Lou. It was a long-term relationship.

When we worked together, it was focused on the practical self-defense applications of Tai Chi. I would cut out the stylized interpretation, which is how traditional martial arts are taught. You go through the formal movement, you master it. You get it into your body and chi. It's very subtle. Lou was at the stage where he loved the idea of Tai Chi but wanted to know how it works in self-defense. He had just gotten into Tai Chi so wasn't yet fully developed in it. He still had that angry side of him, the dark side of him that had to express itself.

We did some light sparring. It was more me teaching him how to unleash his power and how to focus it using mechanics. Tai Chi has very stylized, sophisticated biomechanics with fighting encoded in it. But it's impossible to apply stylized movements. Lou was coming to me with very stylized movements he was learning from Shum's Wu-style Tai Chi. Lou would punch in a very stylized manner. I said, "If you're really in the street, no one's going to attack you like that." I immediately broke it down and said, "This is what's going to happen in the street."

Once I brought boards to break, which was a big deal to him, because he was very hesitant. He didn't want to do it, but I had him break more than he anticipated. Even after he broke them, he couldn't believe he did it. Sylvia who was present and I saw a guy break through his limitations with martial arts.

The force of combat and the aesthetics of power evolved. Tai Chi, in my opinion, is like the highest expression of how it went from fighting—pure fighting, pure survival—into a science and the aesthetics of power. Lou was intrigued by Tai Chi because it's based on thought and balance.

Back then, traditional Chinese instructors didn't teach this. Teachers would just say, "I'm the master. Let me tell you what to do. Do this a hundred times," and they wouldn't explain why. That's the problem I had when I was young. I was saying, "What the hell am I standing here for and doing nothing? What does this have to do with fighting? Why don't I just run around the block? Why don't I just do a hundred kicks?"

I didn't understand these things decades ago, but I'm discovering them now. I'm going back to the traditional way of training and studying the philosophy and really going into the Chinese texts and science behind it. The Chinese were addressing all of it. They have a different, poetic way of explaining things using metaphors. The Western scientific mind is: this is how to do it, just do this, this, this, and this, and you get this, this, this, and this. Whereas the Chinese, they'll talk about, for example, the image of a dragon. Dragons are not real, but if you understand quantum mechanics and physics, you understand energy moves in waves. Dragons move in waves.

They discovered the laws of physics. These were the Taoists, studying nature and studying the "way." That's what cosmologists are doing today. They're looking at the same constellations, same sun, same moon, same human being. They discovered it, but they used a different language, a different mindset to explain. They didn't realize that they were symbols for scientific principles.

When I was with Lou, his legs were so bad, he couldn't kick the way I was teaching him. I was very impressed when I saw the video of him on YouTube, after a few years of training under Ren, showing strength with his leg in the air. I knew of Ren because I met his teacher, Chen Xiaowang, when I went to China in 1984 with Shum, as part of a group of ten Chinese American masters invited to China to discuss the rehabilitation of Shaolin Temple. During that time, I said if there was anyone I wanted to meet, it would be Chen Xiaowang. I got to meet him in Henan because he came to demonstrate, and he was sitting next to me at dinner. That was karmic.

LENNY AARON

Senior student of Lou's first Tai Chi teacher, Leung Shum, and Tai Chi instructor at Shum's school

I first saw Lou at Leung Shum's studio around 1996. I came in a few hours early to organize things and saw him doing private training with Shum. I was a musician and had kind of used martial arts to get away from the drug scene, and I thought maybe Lou was doing that too, getting away from that and doing something positive. When I met him that day, the lyrics to "Heroin," ". . . when I put a spike into my vein," were in my head. When I mentioned this, he said, "Oh dear, I hope it didn't have any ill effects," and he really meant it.

He was a slow learner, but he was diligent. He came. He practiced. If Lou had been out of town, he would come directly from the airport to practice. He was really dedicated.

He loved and was fascinated by applications. He also loved the Chi Gong breathing, and I'm making up this word, but he saw it as magical or something. He didn't say magical, but he glowed. He loved it. He glowed when he talked about it. He was excited about Chi gong and how it made him feel.

Generally, I saw Lou as more mind than body. He wasn't that athletic, but in '99 or 2000 Lou saw Shum do fajin—explosive power—on a student. Lou said to me, "I want to learn that." He loved the martial art application. At the end of class, we'd hang with fellow student Bill O'Connor, and Bill would show his amazing Celtic martial art applications. Lou was always fascinated by them, more than I was.

CHI GONG are exercises to unblock and aid the circulation of chi.

Lou had an innocence. That's what I liked about him, the excitement that he had. It's something you wouldn't have thought about him or made sense, but it was beautiful. Just after 9/11, the school canceled Tuesday class. Lou called me Thursday early in the morning, and he knew I didn't wake up early. He said, "Please tell me we're having class tonight." I said, "I don't know. We'll try. I think so." I was scared about having class. I was afraid of hearing about who died. Lou said, "I can't look at this anymore. Please say we're having class." I said, "I'll get back to you." We had class that night. We talked some about what happened on 9/11, but class was on, and Lou was happy to get away.

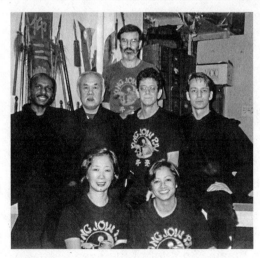

Lou with his training class at Leung Shum's school, late 1990s

EMMANUEL SAM

Senior student of Lou's first Tai Chi teacher, Leung Shum, and Tai Chi instructor at Shum's school

I got into martial arts about 1977. It was right after college, and I started with the Yang style, and then from that I started with Leung Shum in 1979. I guess Lou must have started in the early '80s sometime with Sylvia, his wife at the time. I used to teach both of them, though she didn't stay long. I was leading the Tai Chi classes at the time.

Lou was just a student who, at the time, seemed a bit slow, but that's not surprising. A lot of people are slow when they start martial arts, any type of martial arts, because of the movement. You demonstrate a simple movement, they say, "Oh, of course I can do that." But then once they try, they realize it's not so simple.

I practiced with him. When I was teaching him in class, we would mostly do the forms, then we would get together at his house, go on his roof, and do Tai Chi on Sundays and some other days.

After a while Lou switched to Chen style with Master Ren. I think he did that because with Wu-style Tai Chi your posture has to be very good. Leung Shum talked straightforwardly. Do this or do that, but there were a lot of students, and he didn't check to make sure the knee did not go past the big toe. Lou had a lot of knee problems, and even before he got to know Ren, I would give him books on knees. He said when he studied Chen style, he didn't have any knee problems.

Lou was very motivated to learn. He found it valuable. It could be generalized for all of Tai Chi [that] basically the breathing is very important, because you move with the breath. So a lot of the exercises start by breathing. With Wu style, if you just walked in off the street, we teach you how to breathe, breathe with the movement, how to walk with the breathing. When you walk, you move with the breath and you really gain a control of not only your emotions but your physical actions.

You learn how to move with the breath. When you're moving with the breath, it means if you breathe slowly, you move slowly. If you breathe fast, you move fast. By learning to control your breath, [in] any situation where there's a lot of stress you will tend to be less stressed. You are focused on what's in front of you. You should always breathe in from your stomach. Diaphragmatic breathing. Leung Shum jokes, "You'll get a Buddha belly!" Regardless of your profession, regardless of what you do, it helps to be able to control your environment and control your emotions in any situation. The breath makes you strong. I heard Leung Shum talking about when you do Tai Chi it doesn't age you, it makes you strong—all of that to me comes through the breath.

The other foundation of the exercise is strengthening your legs, [especially] your thighs. You become very rooted. Once you're rooted you can do anything. Also, the exercise strengthens your arms and your whole body.

At the time, Lou wasn't so much into fighting, because he was a guitarist and worked with his hands. He wanted to be careful to not hurt his hands. In a lot of the movements, you use your hands to parry, and in Tai Chi it's open palm. It's all opposing forces, but even then it can be risky.

Lou and I would talk techniques, how to use some of the movements and such. Tai Chi was his focus, but he really loved all martial arts. We hung out quite a lot in those days. After the Tai Chi class every week, after we finished, we would go out to eat. We'd find a restaurant, and sometimes by the time we finished it would be about midnight. Lou was the first one to introduce me to wine. I didn't like wine. Once he said, "Okay, I'll show you how wine can be." He took me to this one place in the Village and said, "Okay, just taste this." I said, "Wow this is great!" He said, "Yeah, you know, you just tasted a two-hundred-fifty-dollar bottle of wine." All this because of martial arts.

Once he got into it, he was amazed at the strength it gave him. He would show his muscles. With Ren, strength became a focus. Before then it had been about health and mental acuity. Tai Chi makes you sharp in everything that you do.

GREG PINNEY

Original student of Ren GuangYi and senior Tai Chi competitor and judge

I remember Lou asked a question at a Chen Xiaowang seminar. I don't remember what the question was, but as Chen Xiaowang began to answer broadly, Lou said, "No, no, this is the question." He really persisted and got the answer. I was really glad he did, because sometimes people just give up. But he didn't give up; he wanted the answer and he got it.

CHEN XIAOWANG, Ren GuangYi's teacher, is the senior master of the family that created Tai Chi, the Chens of Zhengzhou province in China.

LIZ MCGILL

Student of Ren GuangYi, graphic designer, and calligrapher

I've done Alexander Technique, swimming, and Tai Chi, and have always felt that things can get stuck in your body and that you can process them through physical activity. So when I started swimming, there was a lot of stuff I had to sort out. I was always trying to look for the essence of everything. This was my late twenties, and I found that if I went swimming when I was angry about things, it would be my way of processing it. I felt like I was still an adolescent in my late twenties and I needed to face some things that I hadn't been able to before. Insecurities, boring things, not dramatic. I had been hiding behind a lot of things, and I felt like I needed to step out.

I had seen this video of Master Ren doing 38 Form, and it must've been only after he'd been here in the United States for a couple of years, and it was the most spellbinding thing I'd ever seen. I was just mesmerized. It was so slow. It was so—what's the word—animal-like. I just couldn't take my eyes off of him.

The health club where I started was fairly casual, but when I first came into Master Ren's class, people were very serious about the martial arts, and there were only a couple of women there. It was like walking into the movie *The 36th Chamber of Shaolin*. All these guys grunting and puffing and punching. I'd stand in the corner practicing a form and feeling all their energy. It was very intimidating.

Tai Chi is something I had to work at. It took me over a year. I would make myself go to class. I would finish work and I'd think, *I don't wanna go*, and then I'd say, "You gotta go."

So the first time Lou actually showed up to a class on a Tuesday, I thought, *Oh my goodness*. I was very impressed by how he treated everybody. He was very friendly and down-to-earth. He was also very open-minded, and he seemed to be totally into learning Tai Chi. He wasn't going to let anything get in the way of that. I remember one time when Master Ren had to go back to China and Kai taught the class, and people were getting a little disgruntled. I remember Lou saying, "I'm here to learn, and I think Kai is doing a really great job teaching us." Another time, when we couldn't get a decent room for advanced class, Lou said, "Come back to my roof." That spoke a lot about his attitude.

Lou was really the only one in class who asked questions. He would still ask, even though he knew it already. He was still learning little things from all those questions.

Not every student was a great student, but Ren was so proud of Lou because of what he had accomplished with him. It's the feeling I used to get as a fellow student watching the two of them.

Occasionally Lou would show us how to do something. He was not nonchalant but humble. When he showed us, I would think, *Wow, I've gotta understand this portion. I'd like to be good at it.* It was really mind-blowing.

EPHRAIM KA WU

Student of Ren GuangYi

I met Lou, and one day I had the chance to do Push Hands with him. He was smiling, trying to trick me, and I thought, *I'm gonna get this guy*. Lou was very happy, and you could feel his passion for doing Tai Chi.

For me, I was struggling in the beginning, and I'm struggling now with the different levels. I didn't have a moment of sudden revelation, what Lou and Kai called "flipping." I got to that inspired moment, but it came gradually, bit by bit. I think they're called bottlenecks. We have them, but because of some personal reasons I would have to take breaks from class, and when I came back, I would forget where I was stuck.

Lou in class would show that kind of smile if you are doing something you really love. I think Lou really loved Tai Chi. Every class. He enjoyed his limitations. He didn't drive himself crazy. It's that same smile I said earlier when he tried to trick me in Push Hands.

It was a special time then because everyone in class was at about the same level, learning the forms together. Tai Chi helped redirect me. I think Tai Chi changed me. We are like an empty cup. In Chinese, we say, "It's no favor to be half filled." You want to be a full cup, with full knowledge. But my way of looking at Tai Chi actually is, you can never get the full answer practicing Tai Chi. There is always some new information, you can always improve. You don't become a cup half filled, but you become a bigger cup, a bigger bowl. This is what I think Tai Chi can change. It can change music. It can change people's minds.

Lou was really the only one in class who asked questions.

▲

DAVIDE DE BLASIO

Friend, leather designer, and manufacturer who collaborated with Lou on designs for glasses and signature leather products

My father introduced me to the Velvets when I was fourteen, fifteen, and he took me to a very famous show in Italy in '74. But I first met Lou in 1997. He came to Naples to play. I had been a big fan since I was young. I knew the promoter and asked him if I could go to the sound check. It was beautiful. A sound check is better than the show sometimes. At the end of it, I asked this promoter, please, could I introduce myself. He told me, it's impossible. They don't want to talk with anybody, especially before the show, and so on, but I insisted because it was the only chance I had to meet Lou.

At the time, people used faxes to communicate. I sent a fax to Beth, his assistant, saying I would be coming in December, and I met him here in New York. We started a little relationship. Very light.

Yeah, it was very slow—the best way. We became friends and started working on things

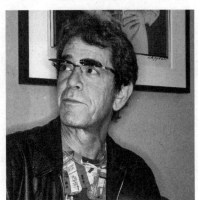

Lou's Views flip-up glasses invented by Lou and manufactured by Davide

together. Our first project was the glasses, Lou's Views. It was years of prototypes, drawings, but I'm not in a hurry, and he wasn't either. It was beautiful because we met everywhere. Amsterdam, London, Paris, Salamanca. Things grew in little steps.

I knew he did Tai Chi, and of course he talked about it, but I never saw it until 2005, when Master Ren performed with him on his European tour. I was always there because of the glasses, because I loved the shows. He was always practicing Tai Chi. Any hotel, any gym, any open place. Always practicing.

In 2013, he introduced me to Tai Chi. It was a special day. Sometimes you have a dream, you wake up, you remember the dream, it was very beautiful, surreal. It was for me the same as on that day. It was June 2013—I went to his house on Long Island. It was two months after his liver surgery. This would have been devastating for most people, but not for him. I found him feeling good. He told me, "Hey, they cut me in two." He took off the white T-shirt and showed me the longest scar I'd ever seen. But he seemed proud of it.

He moved to the poolside and started doing Tai Chi barefoot and shirtless. I saw it heal. At that time of course I didn't know what kind of form it was, but to me it was something beautiful, powerful, solemn, and simple. So I remained quietly there like in a church. It was very beautiful. The movement was absolutely great.

He came to me and looked in my eyes and said, "There is no second option. Promise you will learn Tai Chi." I said, "Next year you will come to Naples and we will do Tai Chi together on the seaside."

After dinner we took a drive and stayed awhile close to the water, staring at the sea and small waves brushing the sands. He started again doing Tai Chi. On the beach. He told me to follow him. I followed his movement. This was the first time I tried it, and in that moment something happened. I felt a huge energy. Like something flowing from his body to my body, from his mind to my mind, and it was something very strong. I think it was the gift he wanted to give me. Tai Chi and the serenity and power of Tai Chi for the rest of my life.

You know, I always felt energy from him. Even when talking or when he touched me. It's something I always felt—I feel it even now, always. There are these ways to connect one to another; sometimes you have a word, sometimes not, but touching and flowing, it was really always unbelievable.

BOB EZRIN

Music producer, worked with Lou on Berlin

In 1980 to '81, Lou came to Toronto and stayed at my farm. I hadn't seen him in a few years, but he had written some lyrics for a Kiss thing I was making, and he stayed at our place. I'd see him outside my office at the back of the

house, practicing martial arts. I had taken some martial arts before, and I was fascinated by what he was doing. He was doing Tai Chi. At least I thought it was Tai Chi. He was obviously not great at it, but he was out in the backyard doing it. My office faces our pond. He would go by the window, and I'd watch him move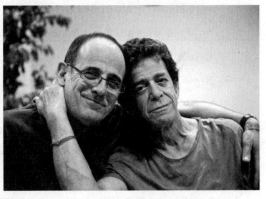

Bob Ezrin and Lou on the Berlin *tour in Italy, 2007*

from north to south, and then he'd disappear. He'd come back from south to north slowly, and was obviously just starting to work this out.

I first started working with Lou in the early '70s. I was just a kid. I'd had two notable albums out. Three, if you want to count the album *Detroit*, and I didn't know anything. His manager, Dennis Katz, asked me to produce his follow-up to *Transformer*. I met Lou when he came to Toronto to play at Massey Hall. The opening act was Genesis.

Lou came out, and he was just fantastic. Lou Reed from the Velvet Underground. Lou Reed! I said, "I really want to do the Lou Reed album, but can somebody introduce me to that kid in Genesis with the flower on his head?" As a result, I also did Peter Gabriel's first solo album.

I met Lou that night, and he came to my house. We sat on the floor, and he had a guitar and started playing some things that he'd been working on, and honestly, I didn't really like any of it. It was okay, but it wasn't important. He had written so many really important things, and this was when he had just come off *Transformer*. He didn't know what to do. He seemed to regret the commercial success of *Transformer*, maybe because he felt it pigeonholed him in a place that he didn't want to be.

I had done my Lou homework, so I had listened to everything, and I was taken by his ability, so often, to tell a life in three minutes. Basically, he used a Greek grammatical device called synecdoche, which is, you take one part of the whole and describe it really well, and that tells you the whole. "Rock Minuet" is filled with that. When he talks about a leather studded jacket, there is just a brief moment where he describes in exquisite detail a certain physical attribute, and you get the whole picture.

To me, that was Lou's thing. He did that a lot, but I wanted to get deeper, and I used as an example the song about Berlin. "In Berlin, by the wall." Wouldn't it be great if we expanded it into something like that? It was a V8 moment. I suddenly thought, "Wait a minute. You wrote that! We don't have to do something like that. We could finish that, which would be a trip, right?" He loved that idea. You could just see his eyes, and you know when you see Lou's eyes when something brilliant comes. Lou says, "Give me a month," and it didn't even take him that long.

He came back to Toronto, and we sat in the same place and he played "Caroline Says," and he played "Oh, Jim," and I just was . . . I'm getting goose bumps talking about it now. It was so brilliant. It was so unexpected too, with all those twists and turns in his storytelling. You think you're going along for a little happy ride, and the next thing you know they're taking your children away. *Berlin* was just an amazing story, and it hung together.

During the recording of *Berlin*, David Bowie and Mick Jagger came to the studio a couple of times. I think they were just checking me out. I was just twenty-two. I was dying. I was fucking dying. Sitting with these three guys who are like gods. My heroes.

But Lou wasn't really himself. He was really messed up. Some days he was functioning, but a lot of the time he'd come in really unhappy and a little fucked up. It was hard to know how much of it was depression or how much of it was something he'd imbibed before he got there, or the results of the night before.

Lou was struggling with everything. He was struggling with the success. He was struggling with Bettye, his first wife, in a big way. Then she sort of disappeared and we were able to finish the record.

By the time we started working on the Kiss thing he had gotten involved with Sylvia, who cleaned him up and took complete control, and suddenly there was this firewall between Lou and everyone in the world. But I got through it and got him to come up to King City [Ontario].

He was in really good shape. He was doing martial arts; he was physically way better. He was obviously sober and concerned with making himself healthy.

Sylvia got him healthy at the very least, and then he started doing some interesting and crazy music. It seemed like he was coming back into his own. Then I didn't see him much in the late '80s, but we reconnected in '93 or '94. We had stayed in touch over those years and got back together again for *Berlin* shows at St. Ann's Warehouse in 2006.

Getting back to Tai Chi, I was interested in martial arts too. By that time he was with Master Ren. I had done Aikido and a Hawaiian martial art called Kajukenbo. It's a little bit like Kenpo in the sense that you learn kata and you learn moves. There's also a contemplative component to it, and we talked about it.

I don't remember seeing them perform Tai Chi onstage while touring, but I do remember Ren and others putting on the little show for him on his seventieth birthday. That was cool. It was a great night. It truly was like he stepped into an alternate reality. He comes into this little theater, and he was being a little grouchy about it, coming down the stairs, and

KATA is the Japanese term for the choreographed routines created to teach technical knowledge and train the body.

then he started to realize. It's like: *This is your life, Lou Reed.* Everybody in every seat was somebody he knew, and it really tweaked his head. He wore a crown. He said he loved me, and I felt that he did, and I loved him. It was clear.

BILL BENTLEY

Friend who worked with Lou as his label representative at Sire and Warner Bros. Records

I think Lou knew that it was a long game, and he was going to keep creating. I think when he really started doing Tai Chi more seriously, that really fueled his creativity, because he became so strong. He used to put out his arm and go, like, "Feel that, Billy man. That's a lethal weapon."

With the Tai Chi, Lou had an intensity of focus and kind of obsession with things that really interested him. It almost was one thing. He felt like he was in a whole new area once he got into the Tai Chi completely with Master Ren.

In 2008, we went down to Austin, and Lou was the keynote speaker at South by Southwest. Lou had a nice room at the Four Seasons, but he needed an area to practice with his swords. I said to the concierge desk, "Lou needs a big room. He's going to be swinging these big swords, and he needs privacy." The concierge says, "Well, he could do it out on the lawn." I said, "No, no, no. He can't do it out on the lawn." The concierge started laughing like we were kidding him. Lou was standing behind and gave the guy that look. And the concierge broke out in a sweat, looked at me, and got Lou the room.

Tai Chi was like a lifeline to him. I think he really needed to practice before he did a show. In 2004, when we recorded *Animal Serenade* live in Los Angeles, Master Ren was there onstage with Lou and the band. Lou made sure when we did the photo layout that there was a picture with him. He was like, "We have to have that picture. We really have to have that picture." It was such a part of Lou, the Tai Chi.

One of our last times together in LA, he came out to do some press. I forget what it was for, but we were riding around in the town car. You know, not a stretch, but a town car, and we started talking. I was starting to develop something called post-polio syndrome. I was telling Lou about it, how my body was seizing up on me. He said, "Well, you have to do Tai Chi. Here, let me give you a lesson." He was giving me a lesson in the back of this car I clearly couldn't do, but he wouldn't stop. "Put your arms there and your leg there." And I said, "God, Lou, can we do this somewhere when we're not in a car?"

Sometimes in your life you just have this little moment when you're really ready for somebody to teach you. That happened when we met. Lou believed in me. Whenever I have any doubts, I think, *What would Lou say? What would Lou do?* I can feel him kind of next to me. It's a connection that is so unique and wonderful. He was like an astronaut who was the first one out in space. From day one and from when he was a teenager, he went first. A lot of times he got the glory. A lot of times he paid the price, but not for one second did it ever stop him. That was the beauty of it. Most artists I worked with, you'd hear, "Well, that last one didn't work. How are we going to change things so this one will succeed?" Lou never said that.

BRAD HAMPTON

Manager in early '00s of Canal Street Communications, Laurie Anderson's studio

The first time I met Lou was actually at Mass MoCA. It was September 2004 and was the second week I was working at Canal Street.

I have such specific memories of Lou. He was so eagle-eyed. He saw everything. He would sit on the couch, and people would be coming and going, and he had a way—he could tell in one second what was going on, and you would know immediately what he thought. He was clear and didn't filter anything. It was comforting for me. I was never confused when to talk to him. It was instantly clear.

I met Ren about 2007. It's crazy but I never saw Lou do Tai Chi. I would call his assistant about something and it was always, "Lou's on the roof." He was always on the roof. It's hard to believe I never saw it. It's amazing now, just watching videos of him doing Tai Chi. But by 2010 he was becoming more ill. It was a very tough time. That laser focus was dulled. He began practicing Tai Chi more and more. You could tell that it was grounding him. I think it became something more than a passionate hobby; it became what he did to survive.

I only saw how cruel he could be a couple of times. I was protected by the Laurie/Canal Street umbrella, but I heard about it from his assistants. What I saw was perfectionism and impatience, never random cruelty. In the seven years I worked at Canal Street, Lou went through sixteen assistants. For me, again, I felt like I was completely protected. He was not going to mess with Canal Street.

What I saw was the humor and gentleness. He was searingly funny and so sharp. But if you ask most strangers, those would not be the terms they would use to define Lou. The whole caricature of him is so bizarre to me. Maybe the intense wall he built between himself and the media was completely misunderstood.

God, I never wanted to disappoint him. I found that the one time I did, I was just like, *Shit, that just felt so bad*. You wanted to be your best self for him because he was giving that to you. He was a good friend. He was true to every one of us. You got all of him. There was no half Lou. It was one hundred percent Lou, so to disappoint him, to me, was the worst thing that could ever happen. Once you earned it, he placed a lot of trust in you.

PRISCILLA POLLEY

Lou's personal assistant

I started working with Lou in 2003. I went to school for music composition at Oberlin and Brandeis and was looking for a job. The folks at Pomegranate Arts, where I first applied, called and said someone is looking for an assistant and would I be interested?

To be completely honest, I wasn't a follower of Lou or the Velvet Underground. My background was classical music, which was probably a good thing because the first time people would be called by someone like him and be invited over to his house for coffee, randomly, it would be pretty intense. But for me, it was pretty straightforward. I went over to 11th Street and we talked, and he was like, "Great." I went to Brandeis. You know, I joked that I was basically hired for going to a good Jewish-supporting school. And then I started working right away.

I just remember Tai Chi was a big part of my experience with Lou. That was always a fundamental thing he did. My husband at the time did Tai Chi, and through pure coincidence he studied with Master Ren too.

My experience with Lou doing Tai Chi was that he was extremely playful with it, and that was the difference between his interpretation of Tai Chi and what I was used to. He did Tai Chi as a playful activity and a very joyful activity.

When Master Ren came to 11th Street, they would be doing their thing. And they would either be in the house or on the roof. Sometimes the practice would turn into games of tag. I recall being used as a human shield at one point, between Ren and Lou on some sort of tag-oriented activity. So it was more than Tai Chi. It was actually a very joyful interaction that had a lot of freedom in it.

They were like brothers; they had a lot of respect for each other. Neither seemed to dominate the other. They each brought different things to the relationship.

I'd heard that Lou could be difficult. He knew that he had negative be-haviors and energies that he was trying to stop. He told me on more than one occasion, "I don't want to yell at you. If I ever yell at you, just walk away from me. Just walk away or tell me to shut the fuck up, and just walk out the door."

You know what? He never really yelled at me, and I had a really good relationship with him. I saw him get angry and yell at other people, and I learned from talking with him that Tai Chi and also meditation were the ways of trying to tackle that demon.

Another thing about Lou: When I was thirteen I had arthritis in my feet and was supposed to have surgery, which I still haven't done. Lou would always say, "Your shoes!" He'd lecture me. "You have feet problems. Your shoes are going to kill your feet. They need to be flexible. You can't move properly." He would go on and on about this shoe thing. And then one day, "I can't take it anymore. I just cannot take your shoes anymore. I need to buy you new shoes because this is just not okay. You're going to hurt your-self. These boots, they're too heavy. We're going to go buy shoes." Lou put me in the car and we went to Comme des Garçons to buy sneakers.

When I stopped working for him, we both cried. I thought, *I got to get out of here, because everybody's crying*. I left. It was super emotional to me, super emotional for him. For three years I spent all my time with this person, and I still say he was probably the nicest boss I ever had.

ANNIE OHAYON

Friend and Lou's publicist from the mid-1990s to 2000s

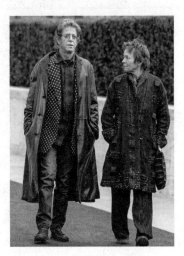

With Lou, I don't think any of the things he would have done, whether the food or Tai Chi, would have happened if he was not also motivated and capable of just getting up and doing it.

That, I inherited . . . I mean I always had dis-cipline, but I inherited that in a way from him. Even with the smallest problem, he'd say you've got to treat it with the utmost discipline and importance.

With respect to his Tai Chi practice, it was also beneficial for me to make sure it happened; other-wise he wouldn't do interviews with journalists.

Lou with Laurie Anderson at the Metropolitan Opera 125th anniversary gala at Lincoln Center, March 2009

I remember one time when Lou was on one of those diets when we went to France for a photo exhibit. So we arrived late at the castle where we were staying, and our hosts served us mozzarella, tomato, and green salad. Lou said, "I told you I need to eat light." I said, "But this is light." He said, "But I need a hamburger. I need to have some meat." So they found some duck and then he was happy. Those were the things that were going on with food when he was on tour.

SCOTT RICHMAN: For fun, we used to call Lou the Larry David of rock and roll. Do you remember the Larry David show that he loved so much?

ANNIE OHAYON: Yeah, of course—he loved it.

SCOTT: *Curb Your Enthusiasm*, because he was so funny. Half of these experiences that you're describing, there's so many of those stories traveling with Lou. It was fun watching people's reactions to Lou's unfiltered comments. He could be direct and fiercely honest. . . .

ANNIE: In the moment, you get stressed, but . . . Not only was it funny but I wish I had written down all his one-liners—they were unbelievable. Because you didn't expect them. They would come out of nowhere, and they would be right on target. Not always very nice, but right on target.

PENN JILLETTE

Friend and magician, Velvet Underground and Lou Reed fanatic

The day Lou came to see our show Off-Broadway, which would've been 1985, the first day I shook his hand I was president of the Lou Reed fan club, which was not a common situation. We were supposed to be meeting as two working artists in New York, and I was actually a fan. I've always been a fan, I've always been someone who wrote fan letters, and Lou was among the top of my list. As a matter of fact, at one point Lou said to me that if he ever met the person who put out the eighteen bootleg cassettes of the Velvet Underground that he would punch them in the face, and I said, "Well, Lou, here I am." When we first met, he said, "If we're going to be friends, you have to stop crying." I was very emotionally taken with meeting Lou. It was one of the biggest things about coming to New York.

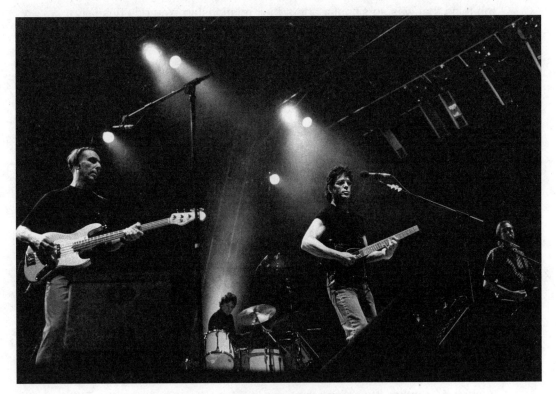

The Velvet Underground perform onstage at Ahoy, Rotterdam, June 9, 1993; left to right: John Cale, Maureen Tucker, Lou Reed, and Sterling Morrison

I remember the Velvet Underground reunion in 1993. Those were very precarious rehearsals. Maureen Tucker was holding everything together, because Lou and John wanted to fight, and Sterling wanted to be somewhere else. So the dynamic was all very brittle; it was all like musical chairs. But that was only between the songs. It's almost like Lou and John had a great deal of trouble communicating unless the music was actually playing, and *Songs for Drella* really showed that. They agreed on everything, except their personalities and their talking. Once the music was there, they had no problem communicating, and that was the thing that was so singular about their relationship. You don't usually see that in art. What I remember being most surprised about was that Moe was the leader and they were fighting, but it was Moe getting the music going, and getting them to connect.

Of course, you know, Moe had raised five children and worked at Walmart, so she knew a little more about the world outside of New York. But watching Lou and John, Sterling and Moe, create that sound, and Lou's sound had changed so much, both literally in terms of the guitar and amp he was using and the rig he had—it was so much clearer, all the muddiness gone—and his sensibility in terms of his vocals . . . the ennui had become gentleness. That was the biggest change in Lou to me. The studied ennui and not caring most jellified to me in *Songs for Drella* when he said, "I really care a lot, although I look like I do not," and he was talking about Warhol. I think he might've been talking about himself.

I think that Lou felt he could be very honest with me. I never saw anything that made me feel differently about that, but with all of the spiritual stuff, whether it was higher power in AA or whether it was the Tai Chi, I was constantly trying to find a physical, provable, falsifiable point of view that would still allow me to respect everything he was getting from it, because the positives of this were manifest. It was wonderful for his physical fitness. Lou tended to have a mind that went very, very quickly, and he was discovering, as I have getting older, the benefits of being able to have some peace and emptiness in one's mind. To have some control over being able to see consciousness as different from thoughts, and the self as different from thoughts.

Lou would talk about things that he felt spiritual about, and then I would digest those in a way that was nonspiritual and then spit that back to him, and then he would digest that and put it through, and we would go back and forth. I've used, as we've talked, the word "supernatural" and the word "spiritual," and neither of those is adequate. "Falsifiable," "objective" are two other words, and Lou and I danced around that, and there's no doubt that the conversations I had with Lou in the early '90s came back to me in the mid-2010s in looking out for mindfulness, and certainly made me more open to Sam Harris [philosopher, author, and podcaster] to talk to me about that. But I know that there's a lot of people in the Sam Harris school that practiced Tai Chi in a totally secular way. So, boy, do I want to tell you that Lou practiced Tai Chi in a nonspiritual, secular way, and, boy, do I know that's wrong.

So when Lou was using magic, like in *Magic and Loss*, or the many other times he used magic, he used it very differently from my use, although when he said in "Dirty Blvd.," "He's found a book on magic in a garbage can," he referred to my kind of magic, and the trickery of that. I'm one of the magicians who embraces the word "tricks." I think "tricks" is the intellectual word that when magic is done the way I like to do it, it becomes a playful epistemology. It becomes a safe space to play around with how we determine what's true, how we determine fact from fiction.

Magic and Loss
by Lou Reed

When you pass through the fire, you pass through humble
you pass through a maze of self doubt
When you pass through humble, the lights can blind you
some people never figure that out

You pass through arrogance, you pass through hurt
you pass through an ever present past
And it's best not to wait for luck to save you
pass through the fire to the light

Pass through the fire to the light
pass through the fire to the light
It's best not to wait for luck to save you
pass through the fire to the light

As you pass through the fire, your right hand waving
there are things you have to throw out
That caustic dread inside your head
will never help you out

You have to be very strong, 'cause you'll start from zero
over and over again
And as the smoke clears there's an all consuming fire
lying straight ahead

Lying straight ahead
lying straight ahead
As the smoke clears there's an all consuming fire
lying straight ahead

They say no one person can do it all
but you want to in your head
But you can't be Shakespeare and you can't be Joyce
so what is left instead

You're stuck with yourself and a rage that can hurt you
you have to start at the beginning again
And just this moment this wonderful fire
started up again

When you pass through humble, when you pass through sickly
when you pass through I'm better than you all
When you pass through anger and self deprecation
and have the strength to acknowledge it all

When the past makes you laugh and you can savor the magic
that let you survive your own war
You find that that fire is passion
and there's a door up ahead not a wall

As you pass through fire as you pass through fire
trying to remember its name
When you pass through fire licking at your lips
you cannot remain the same

The building's burning move towards that door
but don't put the flames out
There's a bit of magic in everything
and then some loss to even things out

Some loss to even things out
some loss to even things out
There's a bit of magic in everything
and then some loss to even things out

ELIS COSTA

Lou's personal assistant, 2000s

The one thing I couldn't do is remove Master Ren from Lou's calendar. Tai Chi was every single day. Monday through Monday. Master Ren used to come every day. On Sundays when Lou was healthier, he used to go to the classes too. When he had an appointment, we had to arrange everything around Master Ren, because Tai Chi was the most important thing in his day. "Never remove Master Ren from here, never." I did once; I thought another appointment was more important for him. And he was like, "Never again. That's what's most important. That I have to do. That's my life."

I'm so sure that when he was doing Tai Chi he was another person. When he was himself, he was the sweetest person ever. For him, Tai Chi was like a good drug. It made him calm, made him talk, and it was a relief for him. If I really needed to talk with him about things, I tried to do so after Tai Chi.

Lou laughed, laughed and smiled, when he was doing Tai Chi. A lot of the time he was very angry, but when he was doing Tai Chi, there was no anger. I could see it in his eyes. He told me he started Tai Chi before Master Ren in the 1980s. Once he started with Master Ren, he would take him on tour, sometimes for months, because "I just cannot stay a day without doing this."

During the last year, he impressed me a lot because much of [the] time he was in pain. He was too tired even for Master Ren. He'd be waiting for Master Ren and say, "I have to do this. This is what makes me strong. This is everything for me." I was amazed how he loved Tai Chi. But I could see he was in so much pain, and I used to say, "Let me tell Master Ren you're resting and you're not able to do it." He said, "No, no, no, no, I'm gonna do it, I'm gonna do this. I need to do this." When I started, Master Ren was there every single day. The last year I could see how hard it was for him, and he wasn't able to do it a long time, but he wanted to do [it] if even for ten minutes. I think that's what made him very strong the last year.

I spent a lot of time with him at the Cleveland Clinic after his transplant, and he was disappointed Master Ren wasn't there with him, but a few days after the surgery, he put on the Tai Chi music and did Tai Chi in his hospital room. He was doing it in bed, because he took a few days to stand up. But he was still doing it. It was so important for him. Lou always used to tell me, "Tai Chi is the one thing that makes me strong. When I wake up every single day and when I do this. This is my life; this is what I love to do." And when he was in the room, he would find the Master Ren video on YouTube, and he was there doing his Tai Chi and listening to music. He was following exactly what Master Ren was doing. We would call Master Ren on the phone, and he told Lou what he has to do.

Just the other day I was looking at pictures of him doing Tai Chi, and one thing he used to say to describe Tai Chi is, "When I'm doing Tai Chi, I feel I'm flying over the world. I'm here right now, my body is here, but my mind is not here. I'm just flying."

JAN SILBERSTORFF

First Western disciple of Grandmaster Chen Xiaowang and founder of the World Chen Xiaowang Taijiquan Association

When I was eleven, I started heavily drinking and smoking. And I became a punk rocker. I was a hardcore punk until eighteen. It was seven years of alcohol, smoking, and drugs. I became an alcoholic and experienced a lot of violence because we always had fights against skinheads, and of course we always lost because we were mostly drunk.

I wanted to learn something to protect myself better because of all those street battles. I ended up with Tai Chi. My teacher was young, and the very first lesson gave me an amazing feeling in my body. I said to my punk friends, "I'm going to stop drinking because this feeling is better than drinking." Everybody went silent, and suddenly one person said, "Oh, that's good. Then you can drive the car in the future." I continued my Tai Chi practice, which felt so good, and it really stopped my drinking and smoking immediately.

Lou told me that he got out of drugs because of Tai Chi. When I was eighteen, I was pretty much drug addicted myself, and Tai Chi brought me out of it. I understood him pretty well.

Lou booked a private lesson with me in Germany, just before he started with Ren. I was amazed because I expected a famous person who takes one or two lessons and doesn't continue or is not really interested or is too busy. But he was so interested and asked so many questions. And then after one hour he said, "Let's continue." We had a two-and-a-half-hour session. And then he invited me to his hotel suite. Amazingly, he showed me the twelve martial arts VHS tapes he brought on tour. He also showed me his weapons. He had a long pole, a broadsword, and a straight sword, and told me that he travels with his videos and weapons. I really did not expect this at all!

Chen Xiaowang has a clear, logical system. I was missing this in my early Tai Chi training, and I think Lou did too. That was when we opened up to each other because he had missed the same thing I did before I met Chen Xiaowang. He was deeply impressed with what I taught him—not so much from me but from the system.

I was so happy to see after all those years what Lou did. That he made Tai Chi music and music for a Ren DVD. And that Ren started to perform in his concerts. When he died, I wrote in a European heavy metal magazine that Lou was the most famous promoter Tai Chi ever had. But what amazed me most, because I'm a very idealistic guy, was his enthusiasm for Tai Chi. Whenever I read the story that he did Tai Chi just before he died, I have tears in my eyes.

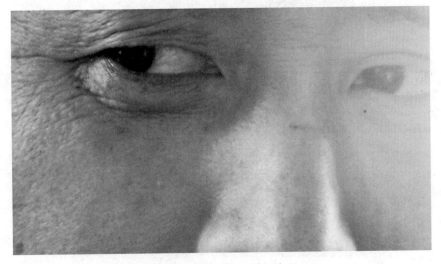

Portrait of Ren GuangYi *by Lou*

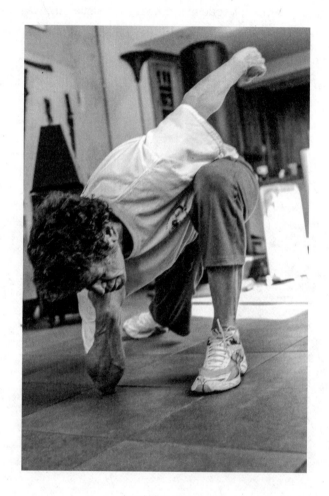

Lou in low stance

CHAPTER 3

PRACTICE

I'm beginning to see the light

Tai Chi Chuan physically changes your body and your energy and builds you up. People think I lift weights, but I don't. It's purely from doing Chen Tai Chi with Ren GuangYi. I do two hours a day every day. Big time. I've been doing it for twenty-five years, so I'm not new to it. If I miss a practice, my body starts to hurt. It used to be the other way around.

Through YouTube we have access to films and videos of things we had only heard of. There is a startling demonstration of my teacher's teacher performing fajin—"exploding power." It's amazing on tape but seriously stunning in person. How can one person do this? Can it be learned by contemporary Americans—people who are not in a Chinese village studying day and night for years?

Size doesn't really come into this or physical strength. It's very much mental and then of course years and years of practice. Through routines known as forms, every inch of your body is trained to be strong yet flexible. But you must practice. The smarter you are, the better it is. The aesthetic is wonderment. But if you only capture movement, you are dancing. No power. If you have power but no wonderment, you are an ape with a weapon.

—FROM "LOU REED: THE TAIJI RAVEN SPEAKS,"
BY MARTHA BURR, *KUNG FU TAI CHI* MAGAZINE, MAY/JUNE 2003

From an interview with Lou by Rob Hogendoorn for "Brainwave: Sacred Science," program hosted by the Rubin Museum of Art, January 30, 2008

ROB HOGENDOORN: There's a very thin line between what works and what doesn't work. How do you determine that for yourself? Is it a mood that comes up, if it's right? Or a sentiment and emotion welling up? How do you determine that?

LOU REED: For me, these things don't involve thinking, thank God. It's very, very quick. I either hear yes or something happens to my body, and that's that. I can tell very, very quickly about most things, whether there's something special happening for me. And that is the advantage of getting older.

ROB: How is that?

LOU: Because when you're younger, you're moving so quickly, you can miss a lot of that. It's like with the Tai Chi: they'll tell you a hundred times, "Practice it slow. Do it slowly." A lot of this stuff, you do it fast, it's very flashy, and it really is fun. However, you're missing 70 percent, 80 percent, maybe 85 percent of the whole thing by going fast. That's just the way it works. . . . No one can make you slow down. I don't know if there's such a thing as fast meditation. That's a great album title for something. Man, I should think about that one.

Roundtable discussion with Lou and fellow students for the Power and Serenity *instructional DVD*

LOU REED: It's a real advantage to do—you're constantly told by your teacher to do it slowly. And the tendency, because we're all living in this frenetic city, is to do it quickly. But if you do it quickly, you're usually skipping over a whole bunch of moves that are the ones that protect your knees and

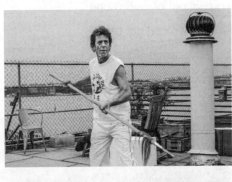
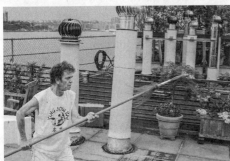
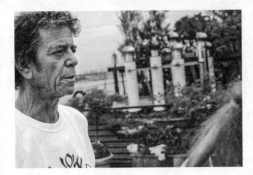
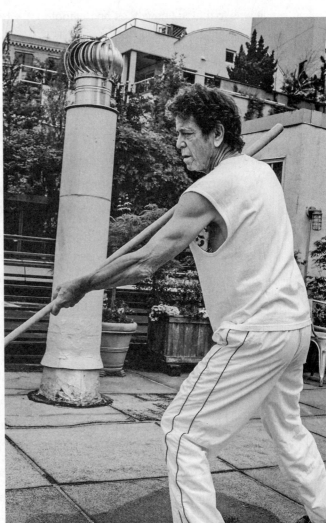

Training with a spear at home on the roof

your back and your ankles. And eventually you start learning from the form to slow down and pay attention. And if you slow down and pay attention, you start actually feeling these moves. For instance, I still remember how startling it was to realize I have toes on my foot that, when you get out of these huge sneakers that we have, that have so much cushioning, when you get out of that, can actually grab the floor. That's a whole other experience. Then you start actually using your feet, and when you're using your feet you're using your legs. And it goes on ad infinitum, but that's because of going slower and learning to be patient through the Tai Chi to be able to focus.

DANIEL RICHMAN (fellow student and pain management doctor at the Hospital for Special Surgery): As a student of Master Ren, I think the whole idea of attention to detail in learning these forms is something that I've benefited greatly from. I think that we shouldn't also forget that these forms were designed as part of a martial art and have applications for self-defense. And that when learning the details of the forms, Master Ren is very obliging in teaching us, I think, the martial arts applications, which helps you understand the form. It helps you understand the positions that your arms and legs should be in.

And I think one benefit and one thing that I find that runs through all the forms, even the beginning forms into the more advanced forms, is this idea of the dantien, of the energy center coming from the hips and how everything flows from that naturally. And . . . a common thread through all of this, and one that needs to be paid attention to when you're confused and you're learning a form, is to feel where the energy is fielded. If something's off, you may feel that it's not coming from your center. . . .

As one who treats back pain, when you lose that idea of that center and where your center is, and when you're carrying something heavy and how you're supposed to sort of bring it to your center, it all ties in, and when you're off on that, you tend to injure your back. . . . This has had major benefits for me, and I try to inform my patients of that.

LOU: One of the things you discover in it—you touched on it—was the idea, if you're moving forward, the first lesson from Master Ren was, it's as though you are checking to see "Is it thin ice over there?" You haven't committed your whole body to the step. "Is it solid ground?" When you absorb that idea, or when you're going backwards, the reverse of it. "What am I stepping on?" This is great in New York when it's winter and icy because in real life you've taken the opening of the 19 Form and you're applying it to walking. Which, right off the bat, there's a real practical application. . . . People slip. Things happen. That way of being, that kind of awareness in your legs, can really, really help you in every conceivable way.

SCOTT RICHMAN (fellow student and moderator): Doing Tai Chi, you improve your level of energy, power, and I think you shake people's hands more firmly. You have a more confident stride in your gait when you walk. You do things more efficiently. Dan, you touched on it—bending over in a particular way, to not hurt your

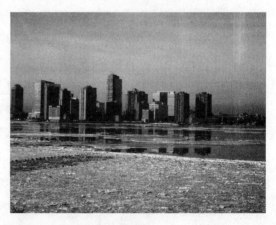

Tai Chi Walking *by Lou Reed*

back. You learn to be more in touch with your body. [*Speaking to the group of students at the roundtable.*] Does anyone have any comments on that in terms of how you become more aware of your body and more in tune with your body and movement?

SARTH CALHOUN (fellow student and musician): I think that you hit right on it. It's awareness. I think awareness of your body produces a comfort.

When you're using your body, an awareness of your energy, an awareness of your potential of yourself. It makes you more confident. It makes you use your body in more efficient ways. And that's the way in which Tai Chi affects you every minute of every day. How you hold yourself. How you sit down. How you stand up, and how you get out of a couch. I mean I remember that was one of the first things I realized. I started Tai Chi when I was twenty-nine years old. I mean that's still pretty young, right? And I'm realizing after a couple of months, to get out off the couch I would kind of lurch, I would throw my whole body up to get out off a couch. Now I just stand up. Every minute of every day it's an awareness of your body, and you're using your body differently.

BILL O'CONNOR (fellow student and Lou's oldest martial arts friend): Well, the thing with Tai Chi is it's actually an emotional experience. So when they say "energy," you're talking about the expression of an emotion, and the energy itself is coursing through your body as you're doing Tai Chi. By continuously practicing different forms, what you're doing is channeling that energy and being able to express the energy, which is the most important thing. Instead of the energy being bottled up inside you, you're like an actor on the stage. You're expressing yourself, and the expression of that energy is very beneficial to your body.

LOU: It's interesting to think of it. We're all very individual, and the expression of the energy is individual as well. But it's expression of the energy that's a very exciting thing as you get to know your body and how to protect it, how to use it, how to use that energy in ways that will make you stronger.

The most fundamental exercise in Tai Chi we call Standing Mountain. Master Ren tells us that when he first went to train under Chen Xiaowang, he had Ren do Standing Mountain and nothing else for six months—that is traditional training. This pose trains your posture, strengthens your legs and back, and calms the mind. Over time, holding this pose helps you start to feel the energy in your body. Your body is still, but your energy is always moving. I remember Chen Xiaowang came to the US in 2003 to give a seminar, and he came to visit the class. Instead of coming inside and sitting down to watch, he stood in the hall doing Standing Mountain for the entire two hours. Why don't you try it for two minutes? Standing Mountain is something that is quite rewarding for both the beginner and the master.

So, Master Ren, one of the questions is: The position of the left foot, the way the toe is positioned on the floor—I remember doing that once when you said to me, "This is not ballet, this is not dance." Can you explain what you meant by that?

REN GUANGYI: Oh, this foot, you know, sometimes it is very up—you don't normally point up enough. You know, toes always are a little bit bent still but not very straight. If you do it very straight, it's no big deal—very straight, no big deal. So that's okay, the way Hsia-Jung [*pointing to student in roundtable*] is doing it.

LOU: Okay, so if the ankle was a little more relaxed, then that would be optimum?

REN: It's much better if it's relaxed, but the ankle is straight and is a little bit tense. It's not a very big deal, you know, and, you know, you turn around, you can feel it. It's a little bit of a problem. It's a normal thing, you know. You're training one year, you're training two years, and you're feeling differently and do the form a little bit differently. After you practice and practice and perfect, perfect yet one time, very, very good, and you want to tell a little bit more sometimes. With Lou, you know this form. I show him and he asked, why I can't do this? I told him you need time to practice, then later you do this with no problem. You need time. Direction is very important. Practice is very important. If direction is not clear, practice hard. If direction is clear and no practice, always a problem. Both ways, you can't miss—they are always together. Direction and practice must be perfect.

SCOTT: Now let's talk about the 21 Form. The 21 introduces some more sophisticated movements as part of the form. It's also a form that is designed to be done in a very small space, so it's highly efficient in terms of how you use your body in the movements made. But it also incorporates fajin in a very profound way with explosive energy. Each of us has learned the 21 Form, and I think we each get something very similar, as well as something very different, out of it. What I mean by that is . . . you could do the 21 really slowly with not using any fajin and still are able to kind of work up some nice heat and a good sweat. You could then all of a sudden incorporate fajin, and then this form becomes something completely different in a sense that your blood, and your energy, and everything starts to flow, and it's just an expression I guess of, a real expression of, just how profound Tai Chi is to a practitioner.

BILL: The 21 Form is actually very sophisticated because it uses an X pattern, which is very unusual in martial arts. Most martial arts, they use a vertical or a horizontal pattern, or maybe a circular pattern, but 21 uses a diagonal pattern, and you're moving in an oblique way, which actually gives you the ability to fight much better, because when you're in a combat situation, oblique movements are usually the standard movements with which you encounter a person. . . . Instead of moving either forward, or backward, or sideways, you're moving obliquely to the side of your opponent. What the 21 Form does is give you the foundation for that kind of stepping.

LOU: The other interesting thing about the 21 is, if you're in a situation where you don't have much room, Master Ren had said to me, "So you do the 21 very gently." You're using it with the stretch—the morning stretch. But you don't stop at the end; you keep going, you do it again. Now you're putting a little more into it. Then you do it again. Now you're on the third 21 without stopping, and you're skipping over the intro part now. Now you're on the fourth one. Now you're going to throw in the fajin and some stops. Now you're at the fifth one. You're at 105 moves. Now, for whatever reason—I don't recall what it is; I'm sure maybe Bill or Sarth knows—108 is the magic number in Chinese martial arts. I studied so many things—it's always 108 moves, they say. Here we're at 105, to be done at any tempo you want. In that same amount of space, and it's the same form. It's just, you're approaching it with a bit more energy. You start it out with a gentle stretch, and you're moving your way up to expressions of fajin. It's really a fascinating thing to be able to do—you can kind of have a system within the 21 Form.

SCOTT: One of the efficiencies of learning basic Tai Chi is that you need no special equipment, only your mind and your body. Talk about where you practice Tai Chi, and the space needed.

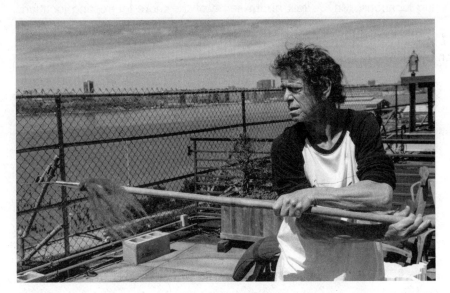

Training with a spear

LOU: Well, I'm lucky enough to have an apartment. I live in an apartment building that has a beautiful roof, and it's all paved, and I go up and—I'd say nine months out of the year—I go up and do Tai Chi in the outdoors. I think it's great to have a great big lungful of fresh air blowing on the top floor of my building. For the winter months, I practice indoors. I have a wooden floor in my apartment, and I have a nice distance of about twenty feet to the left and right, so I can do the longest Tai Chi forms, without doing compression steps. I can take full steps and go from my window all the way to my front door. So I'm very fortunate to have a big apartment. But Master Ren invented a form called the 21 Form for when you're in those circumstances, when you don't have such great space. So say, if I'm traveling and I'm in a hotel room, I will do the 21 Form more than the other forms, because it's just made to do in a hotel room.

SCOTT: Lou, as someone who travels, sometimes 100 to 150 days a year, you've had the good fortune of practicing Tai Chi in a number of interesting locations. Maybe talk about some of the more interesting locations where you've practiced.

LOU: I've practiced in Africa. I've practiced in most of your major countries. Usually, you can always find a park, and when weather is a condition of it, in a hotel. I usually ask them if there is a conference room that's not being used, because usually these hotels have a number of rooms for businesspeople, and one of them is probably not being used. So we just get the table and chairs out of there, and in you go. The worst-case scenario is a little later at night near the elevators. There's always room over there, and assuming it's not Saturday night, you can practice and probably not scare anyone. In the hotel room, I usually have as much furniture taken out of whatever room it is as possible. I'm not going to have eighteen people up there, so I try to get the tables and chairs out of there, and I concentrate on the 21 Form and Compact Cannon Fist. The other way of doing it is—the other forms, once you know them—if there's three steps forward, you do one step forward, one step back, one step forward. You end up in the same place, but you have to know the form pretty well to be able to do that and not get mixed up. For a beginner, I would think the 21 Form Master Ren designed as an application for someone who does not have room. You ought to be able to do that in an elevator, for instance.

IGGY POP

Rock music legend and longtime Chi gong practitioner

I started with Chi gong in late '89. I was pretty beat up, with a lot of skeletal problems. I'd developed severe osteoarthritis in one hip. I basically couldn't walk. I went to the doctor, who said, "Here's the deal." It didn't look good, and they gave me naproxen, which made it possible for me to kind of waddle around. That wasn't going to cut it in terms of what I do. I was looking. I'd seen pictures of people doing Tai Chi in parks in China, and I thought, well, you know, if I could do that, that would be a way to rebuild my presentation.

A chiropractor I was seeing in SoHo recommended a Chi gong teacher named Dongkuk Ahn, who was also a painter and art teacher [and studied with Cheng Man-ch'ing in the 1960s]. He was kind of a salty type of guy. He said, "People expect me to be spiritual, but I like to listen to Led Zeppelin and party." He wasn't a vegetarian or anything. He had a nice unflappable quality about him. I think as these people do, because they're healthy and confident. He had a picture on the wall of twelve enormous guys trying to push him at once and they couldn't.

When I came to him, I still smoked cigarettes and a little dope and was just generally out of gas. He looked at me and said, "I'm going to teach you Chi gong." But he never spent much time revealing esoterica to me. He liked to relate it to the world he thought we were in, so he would say, "Watch rap videos, and when you walk, try to walk like they do, with your hips stuck out," because, he said, that's Chi gong style. He also said, "You know this old dance called the cakewalk from the '20s? You should walk like that." And, "As we get older, we lose the ability to breathe and it makes us grumpy, we don't feel good, and you start wanting to get stoned."

My life was like people who are more interesting, because of being in the entertainment biz. You can do it wildly for ten years and then you have to interface with the horrible, boring, tedious, difficult world of work and commerce. I was in that part of life. I was doing a lot of things I didn't like to do, mixed in with what I liked to do, and doing half of it poorly, which doesn't make you feel good. So life wasn't a ball. But I was hanging on in New York City and touring a great deal, which is very hard on your body. Really hard. My motivation to learn about this started in performance and from a general instinct that I had taken a hit, was weakened, and wanted to become strong.

Ahn taught me **Wu Chi** breathing. He said, "You might like this. It will be good for you." I was in my first class with five women. We lay on our backs on the floor, and he had us close our eyes and breathe rhythmically and deeply through the nose and blowing it out through the mouth. We kept doing this for the better part of an hour. After about ten to fifteen minutes, one woman started moaning and some of them were screaming. But it didn't have that effect on me. I just felt great. And he told me later, "It was releasing their fears, but you do that." He'd

WU CHI is considered a neutral or "empty" state that should characterize the start and finish of Chi gong and Tai Chi movements.

been to one of my gigs and said, "You do that in your work. You deal with your fears in the work you do, so it didn't have that effect and that's good."

That stayed with me, and I still do it if I'm going to perform live. I breathe that way for about half an hour. He always told me, no matter what movement I was doing, "It's all invisible. It's internal. It's all about the breath." He said, "Force it down into your diaphragm and through your nose." He literally said, "Try to blow it out your ass."

Oh, by the way, we're magical beings.

▲

LAURIE ANDERSON: Stephan mentioned something really beautiful, that you were quoted about: increasing your breathing capacity so that it becomes food.

IGGY POP: Yeah, about Kung Fu and Bruce Lee and all that?

STEPHAN BERWICK: Yes, and about the breathing that you've learned, the breathing that you practice is so important, that it's like your food.

IGGY: Ahn said—I never had reason to doubt him—"If I want, I can change my body temperature by a couple of degrees."

LAURIE: That's crazy.

IGGY: Yeah, it's crazy, but I believe that. He told me, "I can put the breath where I want to in my body." I got to the point where I could feel where my bones were getting fused up. If I do the exercise and breathe well long enough, I hear them pop. They pop apart and I get a little air in there.

Ahn was the kind of guy who would drop in the middle of a session, "Oh, by the way, we're magical beings." He was a spiritual guy. I think he was looking at how that magic can be manifested. I was open to that, because when I was in my first band, our manager was an early foodie who taught us macrobiotics. Like a lot of macrobiotic people, we were smoking twenty joints a day. That's not really going to help you when you're eating brown rice! Still, it opened me up to the idea that you could breathe air and there could be an art to it.

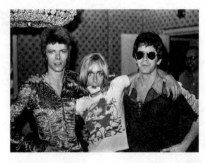
David Bowie, Iggy Pop, and Lou at the Dorchester Hotel in London, 1972

Chi gong kept my attention because, like Tai Chi, the forms are so beautiful and when you're doing them you feel great. There's a grace to it, and it's also a challenge. It's challenging to do it right, but then you feel calmer. You also feel more capable and energized, like buzzed a little bit.

All your functions, whatever they are, if you have trouble with your digestion, the digestion works, and if you have trouble with your humor, you're in better humor. That kept me trudging over to his studio with my osteoarthritis. It was worth it.

Ahn also taught me a few Tai Chi movements. He made a video, and I really tried hard. It's hard to learn that stuff from a video, but he encouraged me. He said, "Learn five minutes of it and do that, because it's different from Chi gong. It'll calm you down. It's really good for you." I did learn it, but I've let it go the last few years. But I'm game to pick it up, I think, when I'm a little older, because Tai Chi is a good thing.

I worked with Ahn about thirteen years. I finally went to Florida, because it was just easier. I had twenty years in New York, which was enough for the person I am. I would see him when I'd visit New York.

I had a funny arc in my life where the full career a lot of people get when they're in their twenties came to me in my sixties, and I just got busy doing everything. Suddenly, everything I ever wanted to do was starting to happen. So I just keep up the Chi gong and a little bit of Tai Chi as something that enables the rest of my life.

Lately, I practice Chi gong about twenty to thirty minutes daily when I'm not busy. During my first ten years of training, I'd do thirty minutes in the morning and fifteen minutes in the afternoon. The afternoon session

DIARY BY LOU REED

THE ACHES AND PAINS OF TOURING

WEDNESDAY, JULY 10TH · WE played a five-hundred-year-old castle near Linz, Austria. The audience here is the same as the audience in Budapest—or Udine, for that matter. People have mastered the jutting neck and sliding head-and-shoulder movements associated with rock—moves that I can't do as my back has gone out.

From Linz to Rome and onward to Beret, Spain, which lies northwest of Barcelona—five and a half hours by car. We are going to fly from Rome to Barcelona and then helicopter to Beret. I ran into David Bowie earlier in Athens, where we were both doing a show. He's playing Spain, too, but is driving as he is apprehensive about the helicopter. I'm trying to think of it along the lines of the Cyclone at Coney Island rather than a Bill Graham killer. It only takes an hour.

FRIDAY, JULY 12TH · We landed on a small grassy hill in front of the hotel, the great techno-rhythm of the cutters pulsating above us. I met David in the lobby. He was watching us from his window to see if we crashed, I suppose. He's been out for almost a year now, while our tour is only heading into its sixth month.

David wears these great costumes. I wish I could, but I always end up in black T-shirts and stretch jeans from Trash and Vaudeville, on St. Marks Place. His wife, Iman, was there, looking very beautiful in a sheer white dress. It made me miss Laurie all the more. I wanted her to see these mountains, but she's in 106-degree Phoenix, in a motel overlooking a parking lot, preparing for her own show. I hope this beautiful hotel has a phone jack that can get me on-line.

SATURDAY, JULY 13TH · After the show, I met up with Iggy Pop—he's also playing. How does he stay in such great shape? I was doing crunches every day, but that's how I threw my back out. I would throw that StairMaster out the window if it would fit and someone else would lift it.

I tried a massage at the hotel, but all the guy did was poke and baste me like a chicken. Don't eat at places called Mama's, and don't get massages at resort hotels.

It's amazing, but the rooms I get on the road are always so much bigger than my apartment in New York. I really have to get a place outside the city. Bad timing levelled me—I bought and sold at the wrong time—but . . . maybe next year. I still rent, which is pretty much how I started out. And I'm sleeping on the floor (my back), which is also pretty much how I started. Only this time I'm looking out the window at the Pyrenees.

SUNDAY, JULY 14TH · We're doing a show in Antibes, but we're staying in Cannes. Bastille Day. We have so many people in the hotel that I got a special rate on a truly palatial room. A balcony looking out on the bay, yachts strewn with little lights lining up to watch the fireworks. I couldn't go out because my back was hurting again, but it was pretty good from the room: exploding trees and helix signs, dancing quarter moons, and tail-waggling dragons. All this to the music of "Gone with the Wind" and "West Side Story."

TUESDAY, JULY 16TH · Made it to Prague in one piece. These double flights are killers. Coming in from the airport, I saw how much building and expansion is going on. And now they have graffiti, which I hadn't noticed before. I hope I get to see Václav Havel. When I was here last time, his wife had died and he was in mourning.

WEDNESDAY, JULY 17TH · We received a tour of the castle, with its tapestries and basketball-court-size meeting rooms. On the Presidential desk, there was a small box with the logo of a well-known rock group—a large red tongue. When they met the President, they'd all gone out on a balcony overlooking the square to say hello to the people. The door behind them locked and they had to crawl back in through an open window.

Havel looked exactly the same as before: open, friendly, inquisitive—the type of man you like, and soon love, on sight. He was chain-smoking and had a bad cough from the flu. We talked about the problems of writing. His: all he writes are speeches. Mine: I can't type when my back hurts, and I have a show to do in fif-

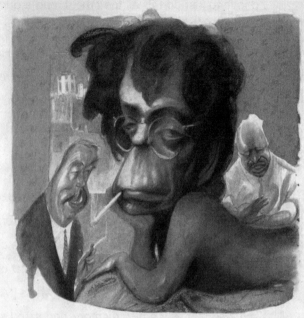

teen minutes. Havel says I could try a bottle of whiskey, or perhaps I might be able to see the trainer for the Czech Olympic swim team tomorrow. I hope he likes the show and stays afterward. But chances are he won't, because of security. We're playing in the old Communist congress; the sound is terrible, but people like having rock performed in this former hall of terror.

Backstage again, sweating and doing stretches. Have to pack later tonight. Havel decides to stay and is in one of the other rooms. I dry off and bound down the hall. We drink and smoke, and he says he liked the show. I'm relieved—I don't know why. I know we were good. It's just that

we weren't as great as we can be. Actually not we, me. I wanted to be incandescent.

THURSDAY, JULY 18TH A.M. · Shampoo exploded in my suitcase and my freeze-dried breakfast mineral powder leaked across everything. I tried a wet cloth to clean it up, but then the shampoo started bubbling. Now one side of the suitcase has separated because the glue is being loosened by the shampoo. I showered, and when I went to dry my hair the hair dryer spewed green powder all over me, destroying a custom contact lens in the process. As I was cursing this luck, there was a knock on the door—the Olympic swimming

trainer. Fifteen minutes and some extraordinary cracks later, I was back on my feet.

SATURDAY, JULY 20TH · Travelling from Prague to Vienna to Zeebrugge, Belgium. Two connecting flights and a one-hour layover. Travel time: six and a half hours. Playing time: one hour. My luggage is lost. An interviewer asks me why I don't smile much. I wonder if he'd ask Miles Davis that question. I tell him to check my inner glow. Some group has threatened to kill the Sex Pistols for cancelling a gig—security is high. What a way to go. Shot by a drunken fan mistaking you for Johnny Rotten. I love rock and roll. ◆

Pages from Lou's tour diary, published in The New Yorker, *1996*

was a little bit of Chi gong and another type of Chi gong Ahn taught me. It's like an isometric. It's harder. You flex certain muscles. Usually for me, I started having trouble in my upper back. You flex those muscles while you hold a position and hold your breath in the diaphragm and then push it out, releasing the breath. It's strong and you get pretty high from it. The ideal is forty-five minutes daily of Chi gong. As I got older and busier, it's gone to twenty minutes in the morning and ten minutes in the afternoon.

I'd love to just do this all the time. I read a quote from Lou, where he said he hopes everybody does this all the time.

LAURIE: He started increasing his practice. He was doing it three times a week, and then it was four, and then it was five, and then it was seven. He was really into that—at least a couple hours a day.

IGGY: Wow, that's great! I never spoke with him about the martial arts, by the way.

LAURIE: Really? Aha.

IGGY: I never did. When I first met him, I talked to him about songs. He tolerated me, I think. Because, you know, he was from New York and I wasn't. But I was okay with that. I never really had a deep conversation with him. I hung out in his hotel room a couple times and his flat once, and bumped into him at shows. He came to a Stooges show at Max's [Max's Kansas City in New York City], and that was a nice memory, and then I saw a very good show of his at Max's that's always stuck in my memory. I'm not sure if it was even a real show. It could have been something that they call a showcase, because there were so few of us. It was in that front room upstairs that was very small with some banquettes and windows overlooking Park Avenue on Union Square. There might have been thirty to forty people, and there was a very tiny stage. He played there with the Yule brother [Billy Yule], Velvet Underground lineup, and they did "Ocean," and I remember "Pale Blue Eyes." I remember he had a very nice french-cut T-shirt on. And I said, "I want to get that T-shirt." I think he got it over on Christopher Street, and he was pretty buff.

LAURIE: Lou was always telling people, "Don't eat carbs!" Do you tell people about diet and tell them what they should or shouldn't eat? Because Lou was always doing that to others.

IGGY: Well, I don't tell. I just watch and see how people do it. It's different for everyone, and it depends on your age and what sort of person you are.

I eat everything, but I do it with knowledge of what I'm doing. Right now, for the life I'm living, I eat quite a bit of red meat, but high quality. In the morning I eat nuts and a banana or something like that, because there's some grain, there's some whole-grain goodness to nuts that haven't been ruined. I try to avoid too much sugar, although I'm aware a little bit of it creeps into just about everything that we consume, including most health food, which is also usually the stuff you buy at a store. It's all been processed, even the health stuff. A banana is a good bet, because you can see it. You can hold it in your hand, you can see what it is, and it's got a coating around it that actually naturally grew there. So I try to make decisions like that.

A banana is a good bet, because you can see it.

▲

SCOTT RICHMAN: What else do you do to keep in such good shape? Even with the Chi gong, Tai Chi, and eating sensibly, you're in incredible shape for somebody whose body has been put through the rigors of performance for so long. Are there other things as part of your regimen that you do?

IGGY: The other thing is what Ahn always advised: to bathe often, but not, like, take a shower. I try to be in water as much as I can, especially the ocean. The ocean beats the hell out of anything else. But even in a pool, you don't have to swim. I like swimming, but if you go to the Caribbean or summers in Miami, you see people from the southern reaches, sometimes older women, just go in the water and sort of sit there, talking for hours. Jamaicans do that a lot too. You'll see the guys just sit in the water for forty minutes, and I do that a lot. It just makes me feel better. The currents and the pressure from the water, it does something good for the body. Ahn always told me to make a daily effort. He said, "Get a little progress every day." And he said if you're tired, do less, which made a lot of sense, instead of forcing yourself all the time. That's probably been the better thing for me. That and I try not to eat bad food.

LAURIE: Did Chi gong influence your songwriting and performance, and if so, how?

IGGY: Little by little. One thing it did was it widened my voice. Like, it helped the low end go bigger and the high end go louder. The performance is where it really helped. I developed the ability to move around, breathe, and sing with a full voice at the same time. It made me way more capable of doing a good rock show, because in a rock show you should be able to sing loud or sing in a way that you're heard, which for most people means loud. You have to make yourself heard against those loud instruments. For the sort of thing I do, you have to use the stage, so it gave me a lot more strength and stamina to do that.

LAURIE: How long did it take to get there with Chi gong?

IGGY: I noticed it helping me after ten years. I went on faith for a long time, and I noticed that it was at least making it possible to walk. I used

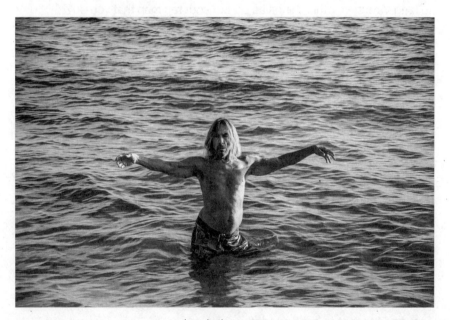

Iggy in the ocean

it in combination with Western medicine. If you look at pictures of me from about 2002, after about twelve years of Chi gong, you don't see this skinny guy bent over. The dude is filled out and more upright.

LAURIE: That's true.

IGGY: I still had my nicks from a lot of damage. There's some damage you're never going to get rid of, and that's that. But I was able to overcome it with the help of this. After about twenty years, I started noticing I could hear the bones pop. *Okay, we need to loosen this*, and I'd know how.

The practice of the breathing and doing these movements, and what you can observe from the people who teach you, gets you in that mood where you can feel that you're actually a human being. You feel a little more human and that it's okay and it's going to work out. Like Ahn said, "We are magical beings." Well, you can be a magical being in a nice, sensible way. That's how you do it.

HSIA-JUNG CHANG

Fellow student and classical pianist

I had been doing Yang Tai Chi since I was ten. But when I moved to New York, I didn't have space in my room. It was basically a desk and a bed. For the first time since childhood, I got pneumonia twice and my health got really bad. My brother said, "Why don't you just get back into Tai Chi? I'm friends with these ladies in my dining club. They take Tai Chi from a guy who they say is very good." So I got back into Tai Chi. It was a different style than what I was used to, but the principles are the same.

I started with Ren in 1994. His class was very different back then. They were mostly martial artists who had studied other things, who were looking for a real master.

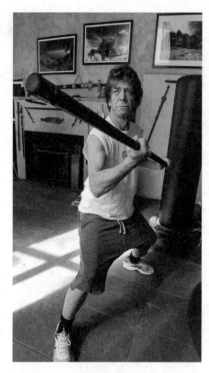

Long pole training

I don't tell a lot of people that I do martial arts. People just think that I might be a crazy violent person. Sometimes people think that way, and you just don't really talk about it. You have your martial art friends and brothers and sisters, and you love the art, you study it. And that's enough. I think people find it difficult to understand. For instance, Eagle Claw Kung Fu is all joint locking and breaking bones. You don't really talk about that. With Tai Chi, though, you can, definitely. There are other aspects of it that are more accessible. People don't feel quite as threatened.

When I met Lou, he already had twenty years of martial arts. One of Ren's students, Lin Butter, invited me to watch a Wu-style Tai Chi class at Leung Shum's Eagle Claw Kung Fu school. We watched them do Eagle Claw and Tai Chi. And then suddenly Lin said, "Hey, H-J, let's do a demo for them." Because they did a demo for us, I agreed, and we performed the Chen Tai Chi 38 Form. Lou was in the class that day. Lou, Bill, and Sam, who was teaching the class. I was friends with Lin Butter from Master Ren's class, and she was friends with Bill O'Connor, who was trying to get Lou to join Master Ren's class. Somehow I got sort of swept into this whole plot!

Bill studied Celtic martial arts since childhood. Of all of us, Bill had actual fighting experience. He and his brothers were trained from a very young age in all kinds of stuff I was not exposed to—all these different concepts that were nasty, unusual, and secret. It sounded very mysterious and exciting. Bill had a different point of view and was interested in other kinds of martial arts. So he read up on a lot of stuff. He would explain certain concepts his way, and Lou really admired the way he did that. Lou trusted him. They were friends for twenty years from studying at the Eagle Claw school together. If Bill explained it, Lou got it. They had a connection that way.

I got to know Lou after class over lunches at Around the Clock on St. Mark's. Also, on Wednesdays we used to have a study group to just try out stuff from class. We also went to Lou's roof sometimes to do similar things once or twice a week.

I found out that it wasn't always safe, but mostly safe, to try stuff out with people you know. For me, a woman who's feeble, it was good because I always feel like I've come across situations where I needed it. If I needed to use my Tai Chi, I would say 90 percent of the time it would be against a guy. So I don't see the point in just women working together. Although that might be kind of sexist of me to say, because it could be somebody aggressive who is a woman. I've come across people like that as well who want to challenge me. It's good to know some stuff.

Lou was always psyched about the Chen Xiaowang seminars. Chen Xiaowang had a way to explain things that was so clear. It's just a few words. And he'd come over and adjust the posture, then suddenly a huge rush of energy would run through your body, like, boom—from moving you just one centimeter. I remember after one, we took a break and I couldn't feel my body at all. It was like I didn't have a body. It was so weird. I remember that. I just remember we were all so excited and trying things out. We talked about it all the time for weeks. But I don't remember specifically what. We were all in awe. It's almost like he had this energetic presence. When you're around him, you're in this magnetic field, soaking it up somehow. It's very weird.

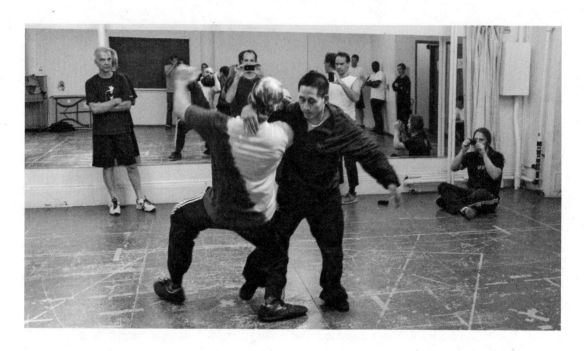

Chen family instructor Chen Ziqiang conducting a seminar, New York, mid-2000s

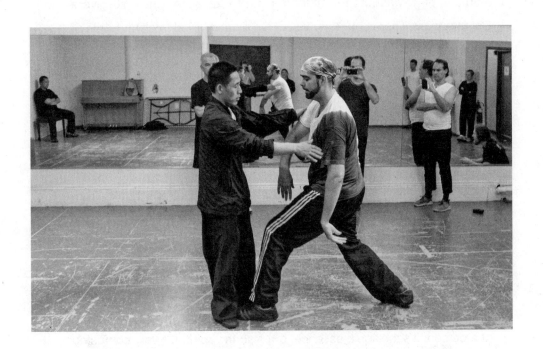

When some of the group visited China, they brought back a book that had a lot of the secrets of Chen Tai Chi. A member of our group gave me the book as a gift and wanted me to translate it for everyone. Understanding Tai Chi concepts requires a background in Chinese and martial arts. It was just too much for me to translate. But I did give a Chinese class where Lou, Tony Visconti, Bill, and I tried to clarify some of the tiniest terms.

In those days the problem with translating Chinese terms to English was the tone. In order to make the tone clear, they tried to approximate it. For example, nowadays saying something like "fajin" [explosive energy] in the current Chinese or mainland China Mandarin, you would spell it j-i-n. So knowing that it's four tones, you would indicate it as four tones, which makes sense. But in the earlier martial arts books from Taiwan, they would add a *g*, because it's like "sing"—whenever people say "sing," it sounds like a fourth tone. So that's what somebody decided to do, to make something fourth tone by adding the *g*. There are other words in Chinese that have the *g* on the end, which means something different, like "jing." Jing is the essence, the liquid essence, of a person. It's the liquid essence, but also the spirit. It's very confusing because "jin" and "jing" are completely different words with two different Chinese systems of spelling those words. This is the sort of stuff that if you're writing about Tai Chi, you have to get it all sorted out because your sources are different.

Lou asked me and Bill to help him write this Tai Chi book. But we discovered that he was confused and horrified about writing it. He said, "I can't write this book." He was upset about it. He said, "You've got to help me." I said, "Well, if you need me to clarify any of these things, I'll do that." It's very hard for somebody who's not Chinese or not familiar with the culture. It's even hard for somebody who's only exposed to one kind of Chinese, let's say mainland Chinese, to read something from Taiwanese Chinese in English. To know what they're talking about, you have to see the character. And mainland Chinese people cannot read Taiwan Chinese characters, and vice versa. Now there's a lot of people who know both. I've had to learn both. But it's a lot to handle.

Lou was very hesitant about it because he felt, "Who am I to write a book on Tai Chi?" He respected the art very much, and he knew that it was very deep and many people had already expounded on it. He felt a lot of pressure. He did not think of himself as an expert in Tai Chi but more like a true enthusiast. He felt intimidated by the thought of writing a book on Tai Chi. I told him, "Nobody expects you to reinvent the wheel. Basically, it's for your fans to get a little glimpse of why you love it so much. It doesn't even have to be all that technical." He could express it the way he writes music, the way he writes poetry, and he had a gift for visuals, he could express it with his photography, just the whole essence of Tai Chi. I thought that would have been a wonderful addition to Tai Chi books. But as it turns out he passed away before I saw any of his writing.

He always wanted to share. He was so enthusiastic. I remember at lunch, he and Tony would always exchange the latest remedies for diets and diabetes, because they were both diabetic and they would talk about protein, starch, flaxseed. Every time we'd go to lunch, it would be like this.

He also loved gadgets and got really excited about new ones. But that's the same way he would get excited about anything in Tai Chi. If he learned a new concept, he'd be like, "Oh boy!" And he just wanted to share all the joy that he experienced from learning Tai Chi with everybody he knew, in any way he could, which was wonderful.

I thought it was great when Lou took Ren on tour. Instead of trying to explain something, just show them directly. I thought that was a great way to incorporate it into his show and put music to it. I thought that was genius. I saw the performance on the David Letterman show and I thought it was great. Chen Village paid homage to Lou, because he really did a great service to Tai Chi. Lou was a champion of Tai Chi.

One of the last times I saw Lou was when we were discussing the book. I think he already knew that he was very sick, because when we were leaving, I saw him look at us in a way that worried me, as if we were parting for the last time. I saw him again at Lincoln Center with Laurie and he had lost a lot of weight from the treatments. He said, "It's horrible."

I felt very honored that Lou asked me to help him out with something like a book. I admired Lou. I have to say, at the beginning, I just thought, *Oh, he's some famous rock guy and everybody is bowing down to him, and who knows what kind of guy he is?* A lot of people who are famous and rich don't behave very well. But he was genuine.

He once invited me and Master Ren to Tibet House for a performance Laurie gave. He said, "It's something very special. You've got to come." I'd never seen anybody do what Laurie did there. It was more complicated than flying a jet plane! Speaking well, playing music, interacting with the people. That was when I started to think, *Well, Lou is something special because he has a wife like this, and he is not trying to keep her down. He's proud of her, showing her off to us, and he's true. He honors the truth. He's not a superficial guy.* Whereas, most of the guys I meet would be very intimidated by somebody like Laurie. He was not. He loved all of Laurie and her talent. I thought it was the greatest thing. He wanted to show everybody. I thought, *This guy is for real.*

He was always very genuine and did not put on airs. I respected that. We were all just Kung Fu nerds. We're just martial arts nerds. We just love all the little details. That's why we always talked about stuff. He just felt it with his whole being. It just came across, and that was lovely.

LAURIE ANDERSON: You totally put your finger on it. He let himself feel things a thousand percent. We've been doing this for years, talking to people about Lou. I'm appreciating him a million times more now, because just seeing and thinking about how he let himself feel that.

HSIA-JUNG CHANG: That was a very likable aspect of Lou. I just thought he was being true.

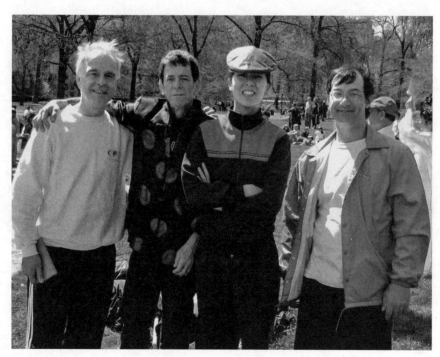

Left to right: Tony Visconti, Lou Reed,
Hsia-Jung Chang, and Joey Bevilacqua, World Tai Chi Day, 2004

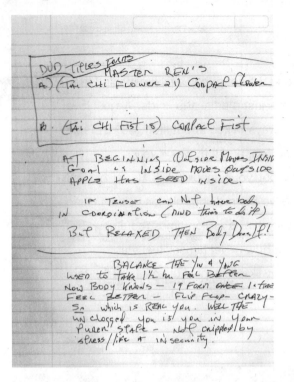

DUD TITLES FORMS
MASTER REN'S
A) (TAI CHI FLOWER 21) COMPACT FLOWER

B. (TAI CHI FIST 18) COMPACT FIST

AT BEGINNING OUTSIDE MOVES INSIDE
GOAL IS INSIDE MOVES OUTSIDE
APPLE HAS SEED INSIDE.

IF TENSE CAN NOT HAVE body
IN COORDINATION (MIND tries to do it)
BUT RELAXED THEN Body Does It!

BALANCE THE YIN & YANG
USED TO TAKE 1½ hr. FEEL BETTER
NOW BODY KNOWS — 19 FORM ONCE 1 time
FEEL BETTER — FLIP FLOP CRAZY
So which is REAL you. WELL THE
un clogged you is you in your
PURE state — Not crippled by
stress/like a INsecurity.

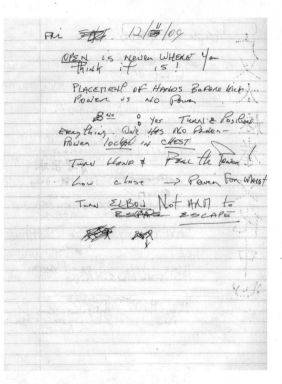

FRI 12/ᴵᴵ/09

OPEN is NEVER WHERE You
think it is!

PLACEMENT OF HANDS BEFORE kick
POWER is NO Power

8⁴⁰ · ° yes TURN & Position
everything. ONE HAS NO Power
Power locked in CHEST.

TURN HAND & Feel the Power

LOW close → Power From WAIST

TURN ELBOW Not ARM to
ESCAPE ESCAPE

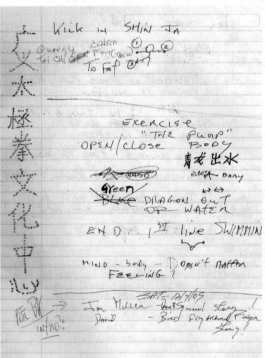

KICK IN SHIN JA
Quingy CENTER
TAI CHI FIST (Green) ① ② ②
To Foot ③

EXERCISE
"THE PUMP"
OPEN/CLOSE BODY
青龙出水
BAISO ELBOW BABY
Green
BLUE DRAGON OUT
OF WATER

END 1ˢᵀ line SWIMMING

MIND - body — DOesn't matter
FEELING !

SAT 12/ᴵ/09
Jim Miller — best Spinal Story !
David — Bird Flu & Finger
Story !
FOR

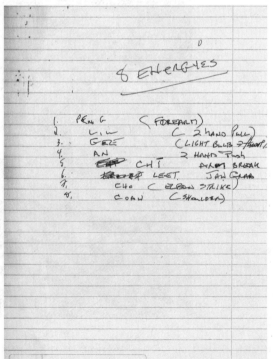

8 ENERGIES

1. PENG   (FOREARM)
2. LU   (2 HAND PULL)
3. GEE   (LIGHT BULB 2 HAND)
4. AN   2 HANDS PUSH
5. CHI   ARM BREAK
6. LEET   JAN GRAB
7. CHO   (ELBOW STRIKE)
8. COAN   (SHOULDER)

Notes on Tai Chi, mid-2000s

FAHGEE

Punch elbows Yang going to Yin
Fist is Yin going to Yank

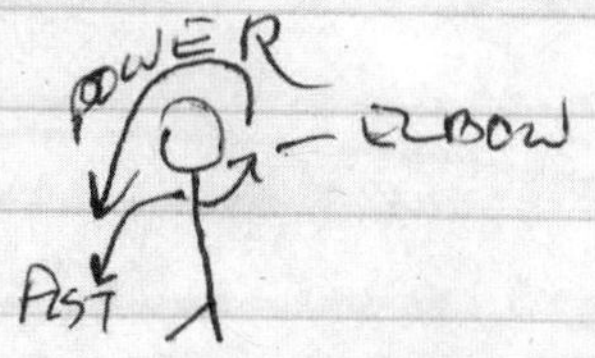

11/23/09

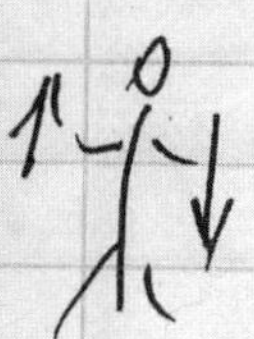

OCEAN DEEP WATER BLOWER.
[i.e. Compact Cannon]

In "21" MOVE THE MOON

M.R. "Follow Fighting →→→→"

[Lock Opponents Energy → Break it]

_____

VED   11/25/09
Swollen gland — do   SHIN JA
                       XIN JA Yi Lu

I did 3 HAND MOVE 三換掌 (sp.)
发动 with FA GEE (sp.) ↳SHIN JA
GLAND WENT down
                       → then
[SHORT SWORD — INDOOR WEAPON] →→

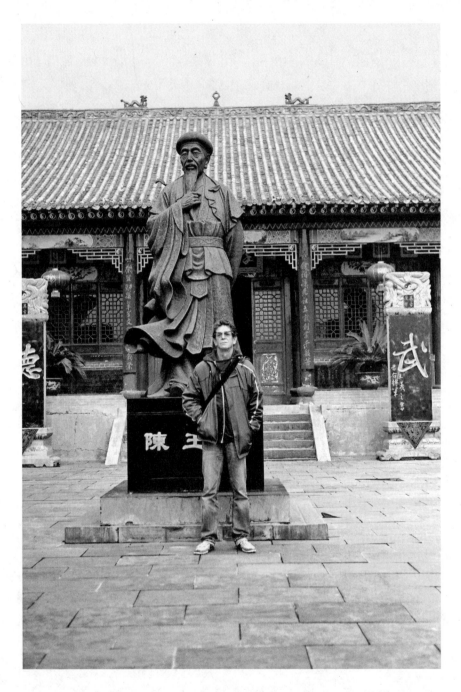

Lou in Chen Village in front of a statue of the founder of Tai Chi, Chen Wangting

CHAPTER 4

CHEN VILLAGE

The earth has changed its course

Chenjiagou is an entire village devoted to the transmission of the art. Nothing fancy. It looked like some old dusty town in a John Ford western.

—FROM "LOU REED: THE TAIJI RAVEN SPEAKS," BY MARTHA BURR, *KUNG FU TAI CHI* MAGAZINE, MAY/JUNE 2003

CHEN BING

Leading Chen Family Tai Chi master, top competitor, and international teacher

I heard of Lou before, although his music and fame weren't as well known in China as in the West at that time. When I first met him, I saw that he was different. He was a man with deep thoughts, but with a calm demeanor and the heart of a child.

I believe the reason Lou was so passionate about Tai Chi is because both his physical improvement and mindfulness were elevated. Another reason why he fell deeper in love with Tai Chi, as he learned more about it, is he had a broad, free personality. He liked free thoughts and other non-restraining things, like how Chen Tai Chi has hard and soft, combining and switching between energies and speed. It's closer to nature. It's free. The culture of Tai Chi is a grand scheme that's huge. Lou was able to connect with that internally.

Since he was so talented in music and other arts, the way he felt and approached things more thoughtfully is distinct from others. Lou was very sensitive to the subtle beauty of Tai Chi. He was able to absorb the calm and inspiration between music and Tai Chi as a martial art.

I worked with a few Chinese musicians, but they were not as into Tai Chi as Lou was. They wanted to make their voices louder and deeper with the strength that comes from the dantien. They practiced for a technical reason. But I feel that Lou came to Tai Chi with the heart to send the art to a totally different level.

He was able to absorb the calm and inspiration between music and Tai Chi as a martial art.

I discovered a new world, seeing Lou and Ren performing together, that was different from the Chinese musicians I worked with, who only touched superficially, at the surface. From their teacher-student relationship, I saw Lou and Ren as Wuxia heroes. Wuxia is a Chinese literary genre about warrior knights. The stories idealize the meeting of heroes and the closeness of the teacher-student relationship. Their personalities matched so well as individual Tai Chi heroes, drawn together by how well the art fit them individually.

When Lou arrived in Chen Village, I went to meet him at the central village school. I then saw him practicing by himself in the courtyard and immediately thought, *Wow, this person is dedicated*. He took no rest, and he was already practicing by himself. Lou's plan for his visit was to learn a form and also practice Tui Shou [Push Hands]. So during a meal, Lou said he wanted to practice Tui Shou with me. I thought, because Lou was older than me, *I'll pay him respect by doing light Tui Shou with him*. Well, immediately when we started, I realized that he was different. It's not like intensive sparring, but I realized that Lou did his Tui Shou seriously—he took it seriously.

▲

After we did Tui Shou, Lou mentioned that the way he felt from pushing hands with me is different from pushing with other people. To me, he was very sensitive and open to feel what was different as much as he could. That triggered his deeper thoughts into Tai Chi. He really wanted to learn more, trying to absorb as much as he could.

I regret that he could not stay in Chenjiagou longer. The way he would've learned and been submerged there would have deepened his Tai

Chi, because it's very different to learn the art in Chenjiagou than outside the village. The whole village is Tai Chi culture. You're surrounded by kids practicing, the elderly practicing, women practicing. There are small family schools and big academies. Everything you hear, see, observe, and think about in Chenjiagou is Tai Chi.

After you leave Chen Village, if you go to your teacher once per week, even if you practice every day, the exposure will not be all-encompassing. Because Lou's stay was relatively short, we were trying to teach him as much as possible. But if Lou could have stayed longer, being around so much here would have fermented Tai Chi far more deeply in him.

Ren is devoted to promoting Chen-style Tai Chi globally to as many people as he can. The fact that Lou got to Chen Tai Chi and became so passionate about it is something you can't even wish for, because Lou was such an influential persona, exposing Chen-style Tai Chi to the world. Lou was such a convincing figure for people to follow and believe in. It was great for Chen-style Tai Chi.

When I first saw Ren perform onstage with Lou, I thought Lou was simply trying to promote his teacher. But later I saw the common points between rock music and Chen Tai Chi, with their crescendo of tempo. Lou must have sensed that and tried to combine the two and show these common points to the world. He was a pioneer, doing that. Also, there is a bigger aspect, or a more grand theme Lou must have had in mind—a bigger level of performance. When I saw *Final Weapon*, the film gave me the feeling that it expressed something from a prehistoric time. The meshing of Lou's music with Ren's Tai Chi was to me very deep and could reach very far.

Lou must have sensed the impact of all these things while he practiced Tai Chi. You sense music by listening with your ears, and you sense

Tai Chi through the flow of chi throughout your body. He must have felt how similar and well matched these sensations are. I think Tai Chi practice let him find a new life, that although he was unable to do a lot physically late in his life, he still pursued and experienced it mentally and mindfully as much as he could.

CHEN ZIQIANG

Head teacher of the original Chenjiagou school and one of China's top Tai Chi competitors

I first met Lou at a seminar I gave in New York on Tui Shou. Lou exhibited solid Tai Chi practice, thanks to his practicing with Ren. Lou was stable and calm, with a good mind and balance between soft and hard. I remember that Lou even taught others as an assistant in Ren's classes. What surprised me the most was how such a huge music figure worshipped Tai Chi like religion.

Lou learned a lot from Ren, and I realize they did something remarkable by combining Tai Chi with Lou's music. Lou's understanding of Tai Chi and how to promote it was great. They promoted Tai Chi to an unprecedented level, because no one ever thought of combining rock music with Tai Chi. It was never done before. Tai Chi also helps promote health, which can even improve music. It shows that the Chinese culture of Tai Chi can be incorporated into anything.

I remember Lou's visit to Chenjiagou. When he came to China with Ren, I first thought, *What's the big deal? He's just one of the foreign visitors to Chenjiagou.* But some Western visitors recognized him, and the excitement they expressed was inexplicable. They could not believe meeting someone of Lou's stature in Chenjiagou, because it would not be possible to meet him otherwise.

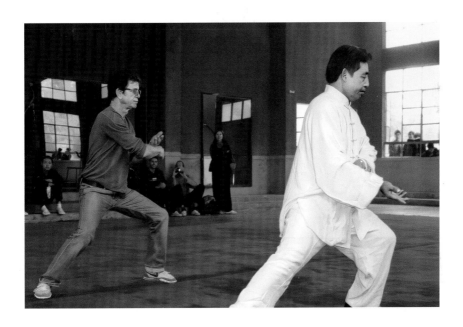

Training in Chen Village with Chen Xiaoxing, mid-2000s

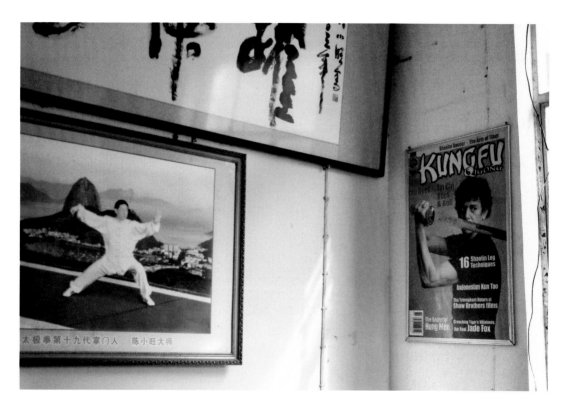

Lou's Kung Fu Tai Chi *magazine cover displayed in a place of honor at Chen Village*

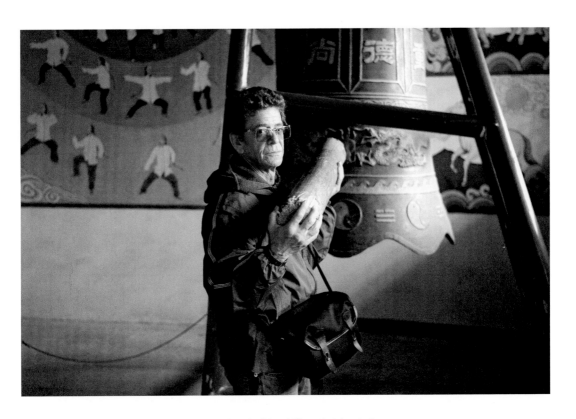

Lou in Chen Village training hall

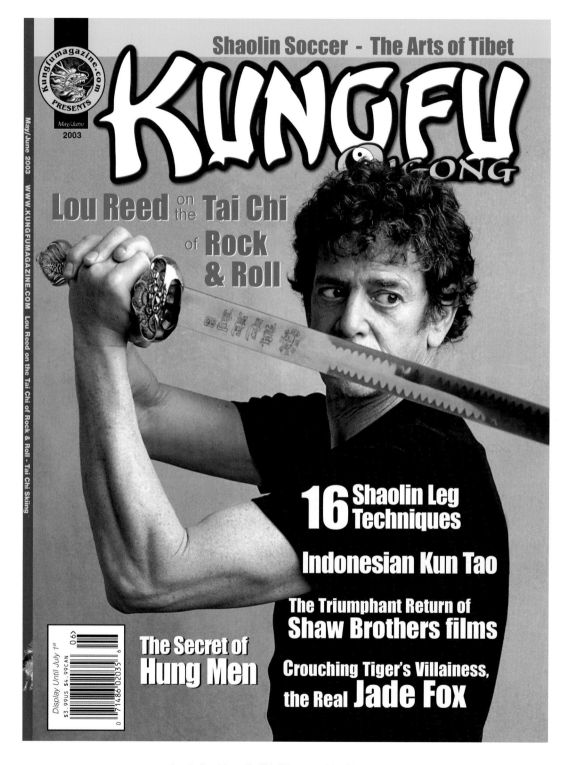

Shaolin Soccer - The Arts of Tibet

KUNGFU QIGONG

May/June 2003

Lou Reed on the Tai Chi of Rock & Roll

16 Shaolin Leg Techniques

Indonesian Kun Tao

The Triumphant Return of Shaw Brothers films

The Secret of Hung Men

Crouching Tiger's Villainess, the Real Jade Fox

Kungfumagazine.com PRESENTS

May/June 2003 WWW.KUNGFUMAGAZINE.COM Lou Reed on the Tai Chi of Rock & Roll · Tai Chi Skiing

Display Until July 1st
$3.99US $4.99CAN
0   71486 02035   6
06>

Lou's first Kung Fu Tai Chi *cover, May/June 2003*

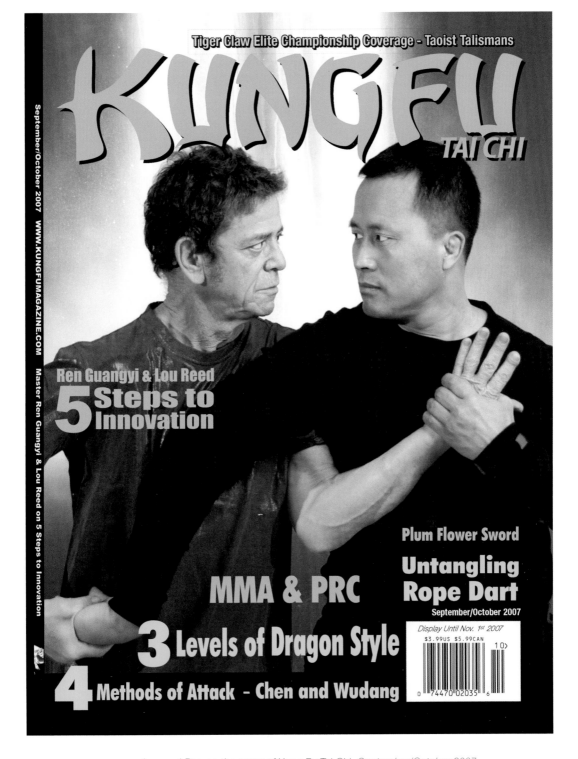

Tiger Claw Elite Championship Coverage - Taoist Talismans

KUNGFU
TAI CHI

September/October 2007   WWW.KUNGFUMAGAZINE.COM   Master Ren Guangyi & Lou Reed on 5 Steps to Innovation

Ren Guangyi & Lou Reed
5 Steps to Innovation

Plum Flower Sword

Untangling Rope Dart

September/October 2007

MMA & PRC

3 Levels of Dragon Style

Display Until Nov. 1st 2007
$3.99US $5.99CAN

10>

0 74470 02035 6

4 Methods of Attack - Chen and Wudang

Lou and Ren on the cover of Kung Fu Tai Chi, *September/October 2007*

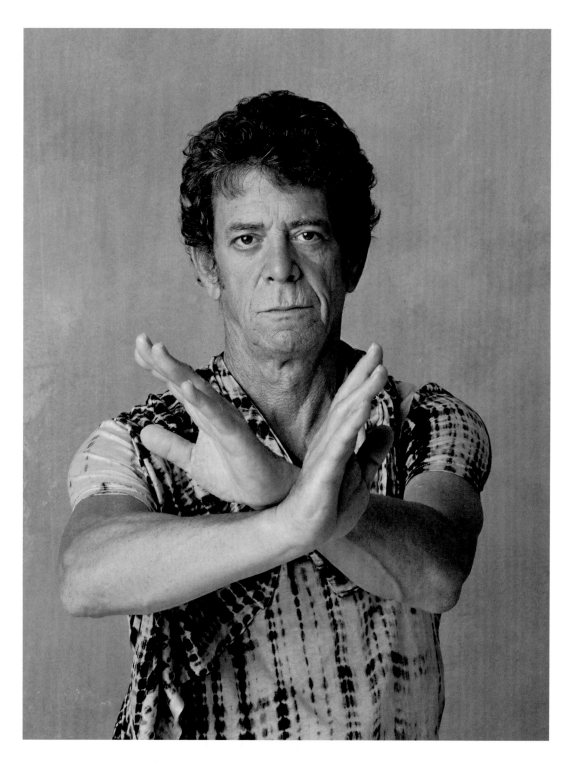

Lou on the cover of LA Yoga, 2007

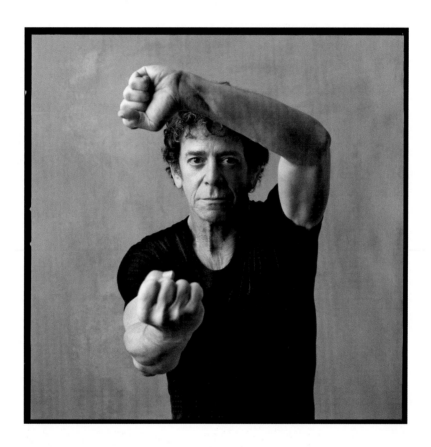

Lou posing for Timothy Greenfield-Sanders, 2002

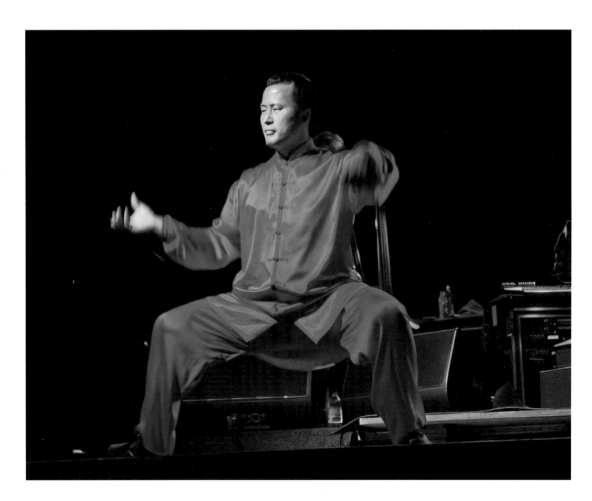

Ren onstage, 2003

CHAPTER 5

REN GUANGYI

The power of the heart

My studies with Master Ren (MR) have advanced to a place I could only dream of and my understanding of the art has been growing to say the least. What MR has accomplished for me is beyond belief. He's extraordinary and I have passed through pain into a new twilight of abilities. To do one thing, one form well, is really the point. Within the form and the correct stance and sinking lies freedom—the freedom to change your energy.

I am not talking about fighting here. I am talking about changing your actual body and its energy supply and flow. It is startling and very real. As in many things, the smarter you are and the better teacher you have control the results. All the practice in the world won't do a thing if what you're doing is wrong and the correction usually causes pain, and you have to believe in your teacher when you are told that you will pass through this.

Never has the motto "No pain no gain" meant so much, as we are talking about anything from weekly to monthly incapacities as you march toward an improved new you. Each correction is painful, as you are being maneuvered into the correct body alignments, which are contrary to where your body has ended up due to lack of knowledge and modern life stress. The fact that these can be rectified, addressed, and conquered is the genius of Chen Tai Chi and the great MR. Practice. Change your energy.

—FROM AN EMAIL LOU REED SENT TO BILL O'CONNOR, MARCH 15, 2005

I had started also studying because I wanted to learn more about power and fighting. So I was studying how to generate power. And a lot of sparring with another great teacher—Larry Tan, the founder of a system called "Dazzling Hands." And then, in my Wu class, one of my fellow students mentioned Ren to me. He said, you have got to see Master Ren. And brought me a tape of him. And I saw the tape and then a friend of my friend's was in his class. And when I saw what they were doing, I said, well, I've never seen Tai Chi that looked like this before and I wanted to learn it particularly as Master Leung Shum was no longer teaching. But at first I didn't go because my friend said the class is SO hard, it's impossible, it's really, really hard! But finally it was just too fascinating, so I went to the class and I met him and then I called around to see if I could study with him privately. When I saw what he did, . . . I said, "Oh my God, a man who can fly. I want to start learning that." And that was almost a year ago. . . .

My attitude is that you very rarely come in contact with someone of Master Ren's level, so every opportunity I could get to learn from him I wanted to do that. So I took time off from what I normally do. And I decided I really felt I was missing a lot of things in my Tai Chi education, and that the answer to it was Master Ren. To show me the things that I hadn't been able to learn in some of the other classes. . . .

Like I said, one of the people I was with said it's really hard. They were talking about the lowness of the stance, for instance, and fajin. But it's not a really realistic appraisal, because you don't do what you can't do, and you learn how to do things. I'm not saying it's not difficult, but it's not impossible, it's a matter of application and the ability of the instructor, which in this case is as good as it could possibly get. If someone teaches you alignment, and I'm not a Tai Chi expert by any stretch, so interviewing me about Tai Chi is kind of the cart before the horse, but just from my point of view as a student, it's simply that Master Ren can show you the relationship of power, stance, and form.

I've found that from my point of view, the Chen style contained many things that I knew on a fairly superficial level from Eagle Claw, and that had Chen elements of what seemed to me the soft applications in Eagle Claw. There were lots of things that I recognized from my experience with Eagle Claw and Wu Hao, and here was the combination of the whole kit and kaboodle, the whole tamale in one. I think it's pretty astonishing. Plus, being able to really generate power in fighting . . . and that the answer to it was Master Ren. To show me the things that I hadn't been able to learn in some of the other classes. . . . He combines the very beautiful form, the great control, the focus, and a really, truly remarkable fajin. When I saw that combination of grace and power, the fast and the soft, the yin and the yang, that's what I'd been looking for. When I started studying with him I realized how much he could teach me. To say the least. So I was very fortunate that he agreed to teach me. And I try to study with him as often as possible. . . .

All Tai Chi has the martial aspect to it, a lot of people don't know, a lot of the teachers won't show it, or they do show it but you don't really learn it, what the application is. I started studying with Larry Tan because I wanted to have street fighting. Not applications that you throw a punch and if you stand there for fifteen minutes I do the application. And you're in your pose. I'm in NY, that's not what's going to happen. So I was interested in some of the more serious applications of it. And then again, I thought that Master Ren's form and the way he taught it gave you access to all these things. From the minute I saw Master Ren do fajin, I thought, I will study this forever. To try and get some of what he can do. And he's a truly great teacher. He likes showing you. . . .

Everybody does something, some people race cars, others collect stamps, I find Tai Chi to be philosophically, aesthetically, physically, and spiritually fascinating. I was told in my fast form there are four emotions you express. I found that a fascinating concept to have.

At what point are you a martial artist as opposed to someone interested in the martial arts? And if you're looking at it that way, you've got a layman, you've got a dilettante, you've got this and that, at what point would you say martial artist? Well, that's a martial artist [*points at Ren*]. I mean, look at painters. Okay, Van Gogh, there's a painter. Lots of people paint, lots of people teach painting, are they artists? No. That's an artist [*points again at Ren*]. A martial artist. That's a goal. I don't think I'm in any position to call myself a martial artist. I'm a student of the martial arts. He's a martial artist, that's a whole other level. . . .

Chen style suits me to a tee. That's the kind of Tai Chi that was made for me, and if I'd seen it I would have gone there. It combines everything. I'd never seen it before, though. Not what Ren does. If I had, then there I would have been. I think that everything happens for a reason, everything happens when it's going to happen. Chen is made for someone like me. The attraction is, that's it, my temperament.

—FROM "LOU REED: A WALK ON THE WILD SIDE OF TAI CHI,"
BY MARTHA BURR, *KUNG FU TAI CHI* MAGAZINE, MAY/JUNE 2003

I've been interested in martial arts for very many years, probably thirty, forty years, because I had thought, I should be doing exercise. Why not do exercise that had a point? And when I saw what Chen-style Tai Chi was, I realized I was in the wrong style of Tai Chi and I should be doing Chen. And when I got back to New York—this is about ten years ago—I saw Master Ren do fajin, and the minute I saw that, I just wanted to study with him immediately, and I have.

Fajin is an expression of power. It's an extraordinary power that you can learn to access through practicing Master Ren's style of Chen.

I wasn't in pain, although with the other style I was doing, I'd started hurting my knees. And I was really worried about that. I knew the school I was in wasn't very impressed with a knee operation, and I didn't want to be one of them. So it was obviously something wrong, and just around that time, Master Ren shows up, and I took one look at what he did and it was so much what I wanted to do. And I just switched, and that was the end of any knee pain, any back pain, any of that.

REN GUANGYI

When Ren speaks, it's like learning a new language about your own body. It's your body but also learning how to feel and identify certain things that he's talking about. I certainly wouldn't have believed you're walking around maybe using 60 or 70 percent of what you could be using, but you don't know it's there to even use it. And Master Ren gives you a key. He's like, "Here, do this, do this, do this." At the beginning, everybody does it really fast. Really fast. But then you do it over and over, and finally you start to slow it down. And it's when you slow it down he says, "Right there—can you feel that?" And now you can.

He works seven days a week, teaching us in our various efforts and classes. Seven days a week, and before that he would practice fourteen hours a day. That's how he got this. I said to him once, "Did you do weights?" Because it's like trying to move a car. And he said, "No, I hit trees." Because I took him out with me once and what we did is go out, find a park. "Put your feet up. Do your stretches against a tree." And then, "Hit here against the tree." Build that up, build that up, build that up. That's how.

—FROM AN INTERVIEW WITH LOU FOR *WE TALK*, SINOVISION (CHINESE-LANGUAGE CABLE NETWORK), 2011

REN GUANGYI

Chen-style Tai Chi master and Lou's last teacher

Lou loved Tai Chi. It healed him, made everything easier. He wanted to understand it and go into the details to get better. Lou would usually practice six days a week, and on Sunday before class he would sometimes practice for a couple of hours. Then after class have a private lesson for two hours at his home.

In good weather, we'd be on the roof. He knew what was best for practicing, like don't practice on carpet. That is very difficult, but he loved working out on the roof at home. He always practiced seriously. You know, it's the details; you need a focus and you must practice. He always wanted more and always tried again after I corrected him or showed him something new.

Tai Chi, like I said, was healing for him. After practice, everything was easier. Problems disappeared, and he felt good. His Tai Chi practice was very smart, very special. Show him one time and he understood. He got it. He was very, very good. He could go very low, and in low style you need a lot of legs, need a lot of energy.

When Lou was on tour and completely exhausted after the show, he didn't want to see anyone. He just wanted to rest. But then after a year of Tai Chi, he'd do a two-hour show and after be very relaxed and happy.

Before going out to perform, he'd do the 21 Form and be ready

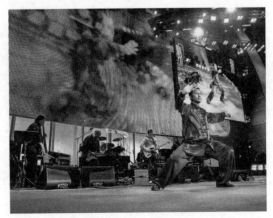

Tai Chi onstage at the 2006 Winter Olympics in Turin, Italy

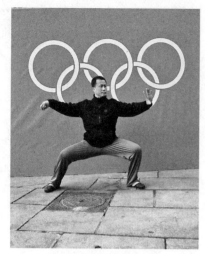
Ren GuangYi at the 2006 Winter
Olympics in Turin, Italy

to go, feeling good. And after the show, he'd do the 21 Form maybe two or three times and he'd recover.

Lou was also a good teacher. If you practice after teaching people, you feel it differently. You go to a higher level. People ask you a question and it makes you understand more. He was a very good teacher. He especially loved showing fajin—explosive power.

He also made up descriptions of parts of the forms, making it easier for students, like Delivering the Pizza. You know, like when holding a pizza like a tray over your shoulder and with the other hand ring the doorbell.

But fajin is what he loved me to teach. It is power that enters from the ground through your legs to your trunk, and all this energy goes to the tip, to the fist. Fajin then goes from left side to right side of the trunk, then hip, knees, ankle, and to the foot to the floor, all while twisting. All the power goes to the tip. If you want to use your shoulder, the energy goes to [the] shoulder, want to use [your] elbow or fist, it goes there.

With Tai Chi, you need to first wake up your body. You warm up, then enter practice, but it comes from the mind. Energy comes through your body and your trunk. It's like an engine, but I told him, "Don't stretch the body muscle—stretch the inside energy. Stretch your brain."

Tai Chi makes your mind big. Lou kept notes about mind and body control and the power. From the beginning, people learn by copying and move Tai Chi energy from outside to inside. After it is inside your mind energy, you move it back to the outside and make a powerful body.

Lou had a good Tai Chi body—relaxed, fast, then slow. This is very hard, but his body could do it. He knew Tai Chi very well and understood a lot of information. His feelings and understanding were very deep. He could do a very low style and his kicks were very high. His fajin was super strong. Maybe he was feeling another part of an ocean. A deep-water power.

Lou said, "We are one body, one big tendon. We have to be a peace-maker with ourselves."

I'm no professor of this, but I think Lou's music, like Tai Chi, had a lot of chi, you know, the feeling of opening your heart, moving your heart. Move your heart, yeah.

KAI CHAN

Fellow student of Master Ren and financial advisor

A friend's father used to be a bodyguard for a general in the Taiwan Nationalist Party so he studied a lot of martial arts, and I asked him to introduce me to a master. I'd always been fascinated by the study of martial arts. I wanted to be like a hero, watching those Kung Fu movies. He introduced me to Master Ren. I never thought about studying Tai Chi until then because when you watch movies it's all about moving quickly. Bruce Lee's style, fast style. I already had a black belt in Tae Kwon Do and also studied other types of martial art, like Aikido. I also studied a bit of quick style, Shaolin martial arts.

TAE KWON DO is the Korean Olympic sport version of Karate that relies on high and spinning kicks.

Master Ren is extremely intelligent. Few can be so successful because you need determination, and intelligence. You also need the physical, the physical body, to do this. Master Ren has all this.

He is such a great teacher at such a high level, people try to mimic him and try to be like a second Master Ren. A lot of us did this, but none of us could be a second Master Ren, because he's a genius. He's a mental genius and he's a physical genius. This is how I put it.

Master Ren is like a gardener. Lou and I were the flowers inside the garden. I'm looking at other flowers and I start to see the flowers grow and start to blossom. I have so much appreciation for this. At the same time, I feel Master Ren blossomed a long time ago so I think he's forgotten what blossoming means. Lou and I blossomed at the same time. We were passionate. We were eating, sleeping, drinking Tai Chi. You have to dedicate yourself to get over the hump. To flip, you need to give up so much. I feel Lou and I had that. And there are two levels to this. There's the physical and the psychological. I saw Lou flip, get over the hump. It was like a flower blossoming. Lou was not afraid of expressing himself, being truthful to himself. That is very unusual and helped him.

The mental and physical thing come together when you do a movement. You have balance in the beginning and at the end, but if you can slow down everything mentally, you have balance continuously, so flipping is keeping that balance all the way through. You gain power, but you don't lose speed. You gain speed, but you don't lose power. It naturally puts you in an equilibrium. Not everybody has the time or devotion to do this.

What helped Lou was having a martial arts background, but he was not dominated by this. So he's not like his friend and fellow student Bill O'Connor, who was dominated by his Irish martial art background. Lou was not dominated by his ego. He is like water. His body doesn't care what other people think of him anymore, he's just gonna relax and do it. It's self-realization of the body.

You know, I remember the last time I saw Lou. I would say it was six months or so before he passed away. I hadn't been in class, but I went to say hi to Master Ren. Lou was there. Lou asked why I didn't come to class anymore, and we talked about my son. I said, "It's not easy to have a kid and then go to class. You have to be very dedicated." I think he said, "Your child is like the center of your universe"—something like that. That was our last conversation.

FERNANDO SAUNDERS

Musician, composer, and bassist for Lou from 1981 to 2009

I grew up in the Detroit music scene with a gospel music background. Lou appreciated my gospel background, and you can hear it on a song like "Heavenly Arms." Lou would leave me in the studio and say, "Do what you want." He surprisingly would like the things I brought to his songs. He used to call me the judge. I assumed my role for the project was to keep peace, balance, and trust. And because Lou didn't trust many people. And he didn't trust himself. He believed in himself. As he was at that point that he was just stopping everything. And he used to talk to me about everything very intimately. I was really surprised. He was really open and telling me about things and the ups and downs in life. He used to tell me that he felt that I was helpful. And it was helpful for me too.

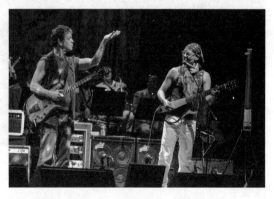

Before I met Lou, I was doing a lot of Yoga, starting when I was sixteen years old. I had a friend that was a ballet dancer and he said, "I want you to go with me to this Yoga class." So I went. We were with this guy there that was

Lou and Fernando Saunders performing

sixty years old and I was sixteen. And I said, "Wait a minute. I wanna be like that guy when I turn sixty." I also had this natural thing with martial arts. Somehow it connected with me. So when I met Lou, that was another connection. He said, "Why don't you go with me to Eagle Claw?" And that's the one I started studying. That was the yang. I needed something more active because I was kind of hyper. Not hyper, but I had lots of energy going out and I needed balance too. So the Yoga was the balance, was the yin. Well, I don't know which one is low and which one is high and relaxing. But it should be the Yoga with the relaxing part and the Eagle Claw with how I got the aggression out.

I think when I first met Lou he had some demons. He was dealing with drinking and stuff. That stopped when I met him. Right before I met him. He talked to me about the whole thing. You know, Lou makes jokes

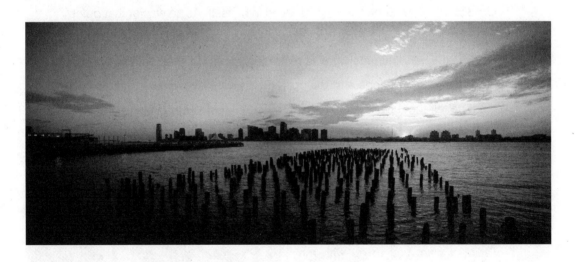

Intelligent Design *by Lou Reed*

about things. He'll make a joke about the worst thing. So when I met him, he just liked talking to me about life. I guess he needed someone to unload these things. I didn't mind because I was a good listener. Then he started getting into the Tai Chi and martial arts around that time. I think he was going to acupuncture or something and that was helping him too. The acupuncture led to the Tai Chi. And I'm really aware of the body, and the body with me is connected with the music.

Master Ren and I were like kids together outside of the Tai Chi. He and I spent time on the road together. Lou would say, "Fernando, you go with Master Ren. He's getting out of hand now." Master Ren was really wanting to show what he can do with his martial arts training. It was good for me and all of us as well because Master Ren is an artist himself.

LIN BUTTER

Fellow student, schoolteacher, and competitive swimmer

I saw a Tai Chi magazine with a picture of Master Ren on the cover. I was studying with Bill O'Connor up in Westchester. Master Ren was teaching a class in Connecticut. So I said to Bill that I want to go see this guy. Bill was a much, much more experienced martial artist. We get to the class, and it's all Mandarin speaking and almost all seniors with one possible exception. So we were invited to watch. It was completely stunning, like nothing I'd ever seen before.

At some point, when there was a break, Bill whispered in my ear, "He's the real deal, Lin." So I started studying with Master Ren in this Mandarin-speaking class, and it was made very clear that whatever Master Ren said would not be translated for me.

Occasionally, during breaks, one of the people, and I think they were almost all doctors or PhDs, they were kind enough to translate a few things. The only thing about the class is that they didn't do very much Push Hands, and I really enjoyed Push Hands. When we did do Push Hands, none of the Chinese men would do Push Hands with me until Master Ren ordered them to do it with me. So that was a very interesting cultural difference.

Lou would come to class on Sunday mornings—not all the time, obviously, but sometimes. What I noticed was that Lou loved to do Push Hands, but he was incredibly selective about who he would do it with. He wanted to work with somebody with some kind of reasonable level of skill. He very often worked with Bill. I knew that he didn't want to be hurt and probably his skill was greater than mine anyway. But there was no ego involved, and I noticed that the people he picked to work with didn't have ego. I noticed others who were trying to get the better of him or best him, and he wouldn't work with them.

On the Sunday before 9/11, Lou and I were practicing on his roof at his apartment building. He and I walked over to the edge of the roof and looked over the Hudson. Clearly, he loved being up there, and he loved the Hudson going by. We looked about, looked at the river, and, I think, talked a little bit about water. Then we looked south, and the view of the Trade Centers was also significant. We talked briefly about that, not realizing that they wouldn't be there two days later. So that was quite a memorable moment.

Master Ren created the 21 Form, and I remember discussing it with him, as Lou and I were two of the first students who he taught the new form. Master Ren asked me what I thought. I told him, "This is really hard for beginners." What he showed us at that time had rather more moves in it than wound up in the final form.

With Lou and Ren it was very interesting because in some ways they were both explosive personalities. I've seen Master Ren angry, and I've seen Lou angry. Somehow they were able to get beyond that. I think for Lou it was recognizing that something in Ren was absolutely authentic, what he had been looking for both as a martial arts teacher and as a human being. I think if you go beyond the explosive personalities at times, there was something really deep and authentic there. I don't know that I can explain it any better than that.

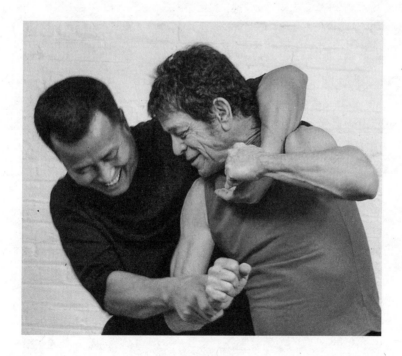

Ren and Lou wrestling

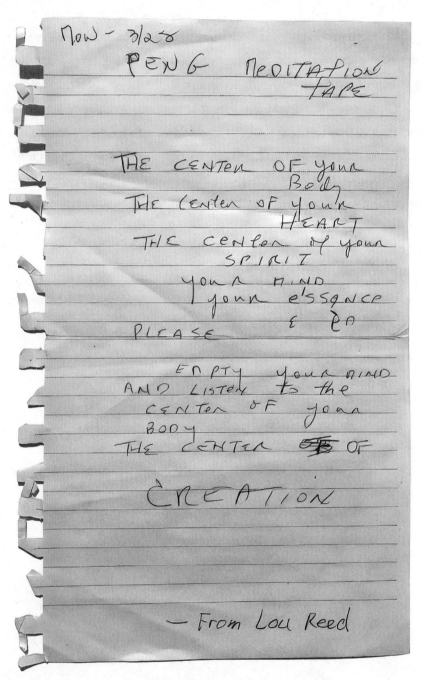

MON - 3/28

PENG MEDITATION TAPE

THE CENTER OF your
Body
THE Center OF your
HEART
THE center of your
SPIRIT
your MIND
your essance
& ea

PLEASE

EMPTY your MIND
AND LISTEN to the
CENTER OF your
BODY
THE CENTER ~~OF~~ OF

CREATION

— From Lou Reed

Notes from Shelley Peng's meditation tape for Lou

CHAPTER 6

MEDITATION

Life's like Sanskrit read to a pony

I'm not a great one to talk to people about spiritual relationships. I'm just talking about the physical body, mental strength. Spirituality is the domain of other people far more knowledgeable than me. I would never advise anybody about anything. . . .

There's a meditation that I listened to from an herbalist downtown, Dr. Shelley Peng. We actually recorded her meditation for the CD *Hudson River Wind Meditations*. But when I put the music out, we took her meditation off so that you could have your own meditation, rather than restricted to just this one that I like. The CD is just something I put together that helps me. And with any kind of luck, maybe it'll contribute to other people.

—FROM AN INTERVIEW WITH LOU,
"MEDITATING ON THE WILD SIDE," BELIEFNET.COM

YONGEY MINGYUR RINPOCHE
Master of the Karma Kagyu and Nyingma lineages of Tibetan Buddhism, overseer of Tergar Meditation Community, author, and Lou's teacher

LAURIE ANDERSON: First, a little background. You were at the Shambhala Center in New York teaching a group about music and meditation and mindfulness. Afterwards, Lou said, "Wait a minute, who is this guy? I would love to meet him." So the next night he got to meet you at a small party. And Lou asked if you could teach him to meditate.

YONGEY MINGYUR RINPOCHE: But he was, like, leading my answers. Kind of like a form of art. Sometimes he said, "I don't get it." But actually, he knows the word, everything. But he really wanted to have that "Aha!" That's different. But then he asked for examples. I think he was really learning from fifty. He looked twenty. He understood nature, and he was really looking for that people experience. He had to have communication. But then, once he did, it was that aha moment.

LAURIE: He made that clear to you. He really loved your sense of humor and your clarity. How would you describe your relationship?

YONGEY: He was my friend and he was my student. And I also learned from him about Tai Chi. I was asking many questions. When I was young, I asked some questions and my father answered from an experiential point of view. When Lou explained Tai Chi, it was very specific and I got it.

After we met, someone told me that he's a great musician—really admired—and that he took a new approach. Once I went to his concert in New York City. We arrived at seven something and we were backstage. I never saw this before. Then onstage, I saw a different person, transformed. I sat in the front row and listened.

Then once I had some days off. He said, "Wow, let's go outside, where it's nicer." I swam in the pool, and then he asked me something about movement. We had a great conversation, and he told me how to fight. He said, "The key secret of Tai Chi is to shield the chi in the body."

The key secret of Tai Chi is to shield the chi in the body.

▲

The chi is the sensation, a sensation of tingling, some unusual sensation from the head to the feet. And for the meditator, that is what we call awareness of the body, awareness of sensation. Actually, if you find that sensation and you're aware of that sensation, that's the one real help for a meditator. It improves your meditation and it dissolves all the conflict of sensation. Your mind and your body come together through that sensation. I found it fascinating.

It is the chi. From the martial arts point of view, it's the chi and then using the movement. For the meditative one, though, it's awareness of sensation. Awareness of body, awareness of sensation. Full awareness. Full basic awareness of the mind, awareness of the body. Aware of the sensation, first, because you'll get a sensation in only one part of the body.

You breathe in, out, fall from, fall back. From the crown. That tingling. We begin with that sensation. And go to other sensations. And this sensation will persist when you have to live your daily life.

This awareness of sensation is just one practice. But there's another practice in Tibetan Buddhism that we call the Six Practices of Yoga. With that, we breathe, and we hold our breath. Then we release. And then we lead, we guide this energy into the center channel.

LAURIE: Using the mala [Tibetan prayer beads] was a really important part of Lou's practice; especially in the hospital when he knew that he was dying, he was using it all the time. What instruction did you give Lou about the mala?

YONGEY: Mala is the order of the end, a reminder of the death meditation. Sometimes we use the word through the mind of meditation. Sometimes we use the meditation to come into the center.

LAURIE: When he was in the hospital, the mala was always with him. He said, when he couldn't do Tai Chi, he was doing it in his mind.

YONGEY: I remember the concert you both did in Phoenix, in 2009. Lou had a lot of pain. And he asked me how to work with the pain. He said, "Teach me." For him, it's very strong pain. I told him about pain meditation. He said he does not feel it. "I don't feel it in my mind, only in my body." He said he can do music and everything, but normally he said, "I cannot do it with this level of pain."

LAURIE: So you said, just don't put it in your mind.

YONGEY: Yeah. That's the operation, looking at the fear of pain, the aversion of pain. Look underneath the pain at that aversion and the fear. And I asked him to work with that. If you do this, you are healing. And it helps.

LAURIE: What are your memories of being with Lou at Garrison Institute when he taught his students Tai Chi? And what are some of the similarities between Tai Chi and meditation?

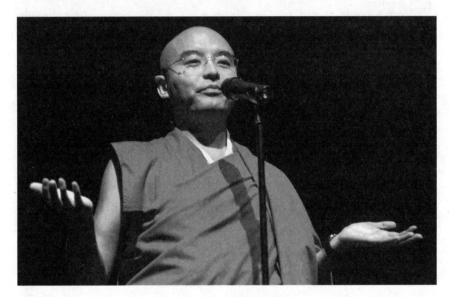

Yongey Mingyur Rinpoche

YONGEY: Me, I thought, *Wow! Movement with the meditation*. It really, really helps. Special awareness of the body, awareness of the sensation. He taught me how to raise the hand slowly.

LAURIE: Yeah. He's pinching the skin near his wrist to pull it up like a puppet.

YONGEY: Yeah. You are not raising your hand. They're being raised. And suddenly, I feel that sensation inside of my hand, and it was warm. I said, "Wow, this is really good for the awareness of the sensation."

LAURIE: I remember him showing people how to pass one hand over the other, and when you do that he described how you feel those centers of energy as they pass from one hand to the other.

YONGEY: And he taught me the circle, the Chi gong circle. He called it "hugging the tree." What I learned is that the essence of the Tai Chi, the essence of Tai Chi practice, is to connect with the chi. Of course movement is important, but movement is not the essence. Essence is

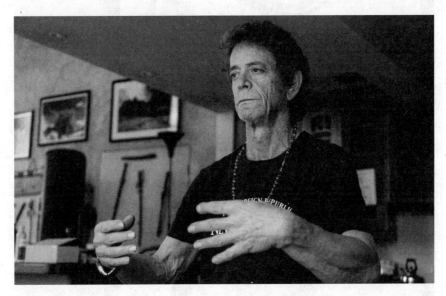

Standing meditation at home

the mind, with the chi. From the meditation point of view, it's what we call awareness of the sensation. And together with the movement, I think they really help. If you really understand the core message of Tai Chi, that's what I see.

LAURIE: I told you that as Lou died, he was completely conscious. And he was doing Cloud Hands, a Tai Chi movement, while he died.

YONGEY: It is really, really very important to do meditation while you're dying. For us, what we call the conceptual mind dies when we die. But the

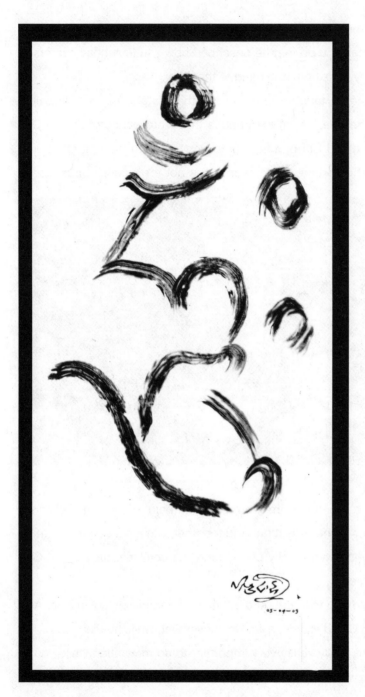

This portrait of Lou was
made by his teacher
Yongey Mingyur Rinpoche. It
is the third syllable of Om, Ah,
Hum, the mantra Lou used for
the many last years of his
life. Om is the primeval
sound of consciousness and
universality and is located
in the head. Ah is the sound
of emptiness and expression
and is located in the throat.
Hum is the sound of the
infinite as it is expressed by
the human heart.

deeper level of consciousness, what we call pure awareness, the kind that arises, actually becomes more clear, more pristine.

LAURIE: Something like that happened to Lou when he died. When he couldn't see anymore, he said, "I need light!" Because it was dark. "Light" was his last word. So we took him to the porch where there was light, but he couldn't see anymore. He was still doing Tai Chi Cloud Hands.

Do you recall the portrait that you made of Lou? We used this image for the cover of the program and the memorial that we made for Lou at the Apollo Theater in New York. Can you describe the meaning of this work as a portrait and why you chose it for Lou?

YONGEY: Yeah. So what Lou told me about Tai Chi is presence and power. I think maybe he's thinking of the Middle Way. It's the balancing. He said that the chi is like yin and yang. And there's power, there are chakras, energy points, in your body. There's what we call clarity and energy. So the moment these two join together and become one, that's the Middle Way. And that produces the flood of energy. So that's what we call the Middle Way. Yin-yang. Yeah.

LAURIE: The last song that Lou wrote was called "The Power of the Heart." My understanding of the portrait that you made of him was that it represents understanding that comes through the head and explodes through the heart.

YONGEY: Om, Ah, Hum—body, speech, and mind. "Ah" is like openness. "Om" is like compassion, possibility. "Hum" . . . there's a lot of things there. We have the sound meditation, which is listening to sound and music and how it connects with you. An easy one. And then there is sound that is calm, without words. Then stronger sounds, with words. And there are all sorts of sounds—traffic, construction. I think most people connect sound to meditation. Sound meditation. It's the easiest of all the meditations.

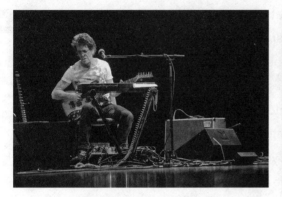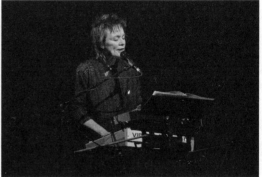

Lou and Laurie performing at Mind Meets Music, a benefit concert for YPPC, Phoenix, Arizona, 2009

Normally I teach a lot of special ways of meditation. When I talked to Master Ren, he said many people think that Tai Chi is just movement. And they don't put effort into feeling the chi. And that is a loss. And some people also, when they feel the chi, they keep looking for chi, looking for chi, looking for chi.

LAURIE: They look too hard, they can't find it!

YONGEY: In meditation we teach how to find that sensation. And then also how to let go and let the benefit be that sensation. So basically, we don't have movement. When you combine meditative point of view and that movement together, you get the full health, you get the full mind.

STEPHAN BERWICK: Have you ever met other Tai Chi people or martial arts people before or since meeting Lou?

YONGEY: Yeah, I met many of them in Taiwan. Some came from China. Before I heard of Tai Chi, I wasn't very interested. After meeting Lou and learning some Tai Chi, I was really curious. So then I met some Tai Chi masters. They talked about the form and then how you pause. And then one Tai Chi master said, like Lou, that chi is energy. And he said, "Form? You can do whatever you want!"

The Six Practices—inner heat, illusory body, clear light, consciousness transference, forceful projection, and Bardo Yoga—gradually came to pervade thousands of monasteries, nunneries, and hermitages throughout Central Asia over the past five and a half centuries.

ROB NORRIS

Bassist for the Bongos

White light bursting into your skull and waking you up.

▲

When the Velvets came to the Boston Tea Party, Lou and a group of friends would end up talking after the show. One night Mitch Blake just grabbed me and said, "Look, I'm going upstairs to have a deep conversation with Lou, would you like to come?" I had never heard anything like it—the way they were going back and forth about angels, about healing with rays of light. That was when Lou told me that the guitar solo with "I Heard Her Call My Name" was the sound of enlightenment breaking into your head. That's another way to look at it. See the speed or it's the white light bursting into your skull and waking you up.

MACIEJ GÓRALSKI

Curator of the Asia and Pacific Museum in Warsaw

I met Lou in 2000, at a press conference. Since I was a popular radio DJ at that time, I was invited to such events. It was his first gig in Poland, and he was very emotional about it, since his grandparents came from these lands.

Anyway, he was pissed off with rock journalists present at Hotel Bristol, except for one: me. Why? Because I asked him only about meditation and Tai Chi, and he said it is not a public matter and we can talk later, so we did.

It was mad. He said, "I want to buy a Chinese sword in Warsaw." I said, "Okay, let's go and look." We went to an army souvenir or sword shop next door, which was medieval knight stuff only. He was looking for a sword, which he used later on *The Raven* album cover.

Since I am a curator of Buddhist art and a collector, I thought, *Let me make a good connection with the man*. I also co-started Poland's first and now legendary punk-reggae band Kryzys, in 1979 to '81, so rock music was my part-time hobby too, or a calling.

I offered two Mongolian knives to Lou, which he bought. He had them at his home, which I saw in studio pictures. I also gave him a vajra [also called a dorje—a Tibetan ritual object used in Buddhist Vajrayana rituals], which, at the time, he did not know about.

He gave me his email and we kept in touch. When my wife left me, he wrote, "Things change"—it was very direct and good for him to do; he helped me.

He sent me his music and books. I also sent him books and gifts. I told him in 2000, "Don't be shy about your love of Tai Chi. You should go out to the people and show it, preach it—it will benefit many beings." At the time, he did not want to talk about it in public, I suppose. He changed later.

Next time I met Lou was in 2008, when he came with his big band for the *Berlin* show to play at the same venue as in 2000, including the famous Palace of Culture and Science in Warsaw. This time we were like friends. He asked me, "Where can I warm up before the gig or practice Tai Chi here now?" I took him to my friend who runs a Tai Chi school of his own. It was very cool.

Lou later became involved in Buddhist studies and practice with lama Mingyur Rinpoche, which he confirmed to me. I like to think that it was that object, the vajra, the diamond scepter—a symbol of awakened

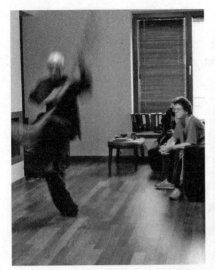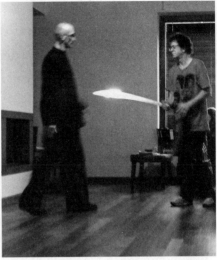

Tai Chi training at the Mariusz Sroczynski Tai Chi School, Poland, 2008

mind and eternal energy, liberated male compassionate activity—which I gave him in 2000, that helped.

When he made *Lulu* with Metallica, I was amazed. It was good. Some people don't like it. I find it a work of truth. The song "Junior Dad" was true of him, also of me getting old, and it was his goodbye.

He is still active from the Great Beyond. My Tai Chi develops much better now every day.

ENKYO O'HARA

Zen Buddhist teacher

Like many people in the cultural stream, I knew Lou for a while. I knew Laurie first, and she suggested to Lou that it would be good if we talked. Lou and I had met briefly at parties and so forth, but my only real connection with him was the one time we spoke about his taking interferon.

I'm a Zen Buddhist teacher and I went through the interferon treatment too so I think she thought we would have things in common because of his spiritual practice and his understanding through Tai Chi of the importance of how the self is present to one's own suffering and so forth.

I came over and sat with him. Interferon is very tough physically. There's memory loss, there's trouble concentrating, there's depression. Something like Tai Chi is wonderful to help strengthen the person. And Zen meditation also helps strengthen you when you're having this overwhelming physical response to medication that's supposed to be making you better. I found him quite vulnerable—not defeated at all, but very serious about this treatment that we shared. I was very fortunate. I had the treatment about fifteen years before. I had the right genotype, essentially, and I was cured. And he was on his second round of it. It was discouraging. Anyone would say it was a very discouraging situation, and yet he stood up to it, and he wanted to hear from me what might be helpful for his mental and physical state. I talked.

You know, Zen and Tai Chi come from the same source, so anything I said to him was resonant in the sense of what was already in him. I talked about not moving away from the discomfort, going towards it and inhabiting it, using it as a strength. And he got that right away. There was no question about that. And there was no question that this was a very tough time.

We sat together, knee to knee, and meditated. We weren't sitting on the floor, like I do. We were sitting on two couches sort of next to one another, and we meditated together. There were a few things we said about the difference in the meditation practices, but both of us were following our breath, the breath of life, and solidifying our intention to be present to what was actually arising for us.

I was wearing malas all the time then, and we talked about how the focus and concentration on a physical object can be very helpful and stabilizing. I don't usually go into these other realms like some other spiritual teachers go. I'm very grounded in the physical world, and so I said, concentrating with the mala is going to help you right now in this moment to be alive to what's happening. So that was how I worked with that.

He was grounded within what he was going through. I think that's a teaching both in the Taoist tradition and Zen Buddhist tradition, Chinese Buddhist tradition—entering into the present moment, whatever it is. And through that, moving through it. And we had the hope that he would be able to move through hep C, through that terrible treatment he was going through.

LAURIE ANDERSON: I remember you leading a meditation at our house at the end of the forty-nine-day period after his death. I really want to thank you for doing that. It was really powerful. Many people had no idea that Lou was a meditator and also had no idea what he was trying to deal with in terms of his health.

SHELLEY PENG

Doctor of Chinese medicine, Chi gong and Tai Chi practitioner

I met Lou around 2002. He came recommended by Master Ren for his health problem. He also wanted to quit smoking and find some relaxation and health balance.

I practice Tai Chi too. I first learned Yang-style Tai Chi in elementary school in Guangzhou, China.

When I was a teenager, it was the Cultural Revolution in China and I was sent to the countryside. We had to go to the country to be farmers. I was sixteen years old. I wanted to study, but schools were all closed, so the kids mostly went to work on farms. I worked in the field maybe thirteen hours a day during the season. I became very sick. I had hepatitis. Even though I had this, I was still needed as a worker. Tai Chi and Chi gong saved my life.

During the Cultural Revolution, they threw everything out. In bookstores and libraries, you couldn't get any books about Chi gong. My neighbor had been very sick, and she learned Chi gong. I was about eighteen years old, and I went to a neighbor to ask her if she would teach me Chi gong. She gave me a very thin book about Chi gong and said, "You read that." I read it and made a copy by hand. I still have that book.

Later I learned Chinese medicine, but I know how important it is for people to use self-healing. It's more important than any medicine. Using self-healing, you inhale and think . . . *Quiet.* With inhalation, the chi goes down. You accept the chi to quiet your mind. When you exhale, you slowly lose your whole body. Just this simple. This is self-healing.

I would describe this to Lou, and every time he came for acupuncture, he'd ask for a meditation. Every time. I did a combined treatment. Acupuncture, acupressure, sometimes the beads. During acupressure I practiced meditation with him. He was a special patient to me.

I would massage his head, his body, at the time I say, "Release. Relax. Aware. Relax. Aware." And then, he was just in a different world.

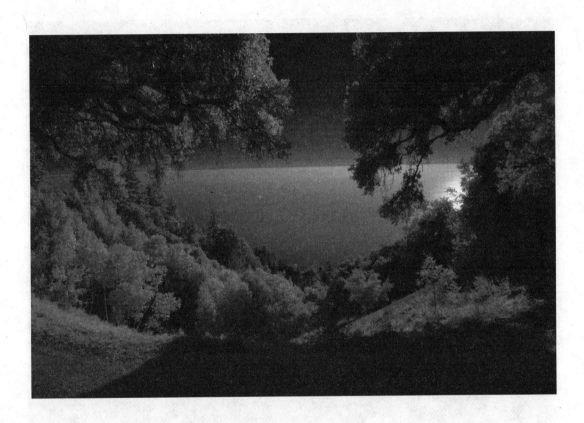

Big Sur, CA *by Lou Reed*

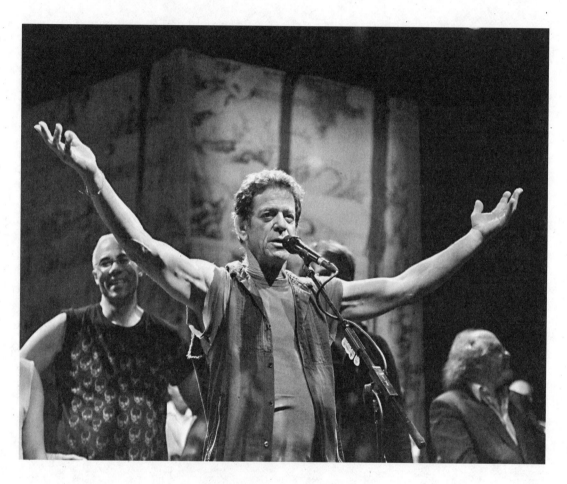

Lou onstage, Berlin tour, Rome, 2007

CHAPTER 7

TAI CHI IN ART

Caught between the twisted stars,
the plotted lines the faulty map

Something I wanted to do for a long time: put Tai Chi to music. But you have to find a master as skilled as Ren, who not only has the martial talent but the feeling too. Ren doesn't just do a chunk of the form. He creates a different performance every night—what he feels like, what he feels suits the music. And his sense of timing is flawless; we never need to cue him. You couldn't just put any Tai Chi guy up there. It wouldn't work. It has to be a real master like Ren. There's no one like him, no one I've seen of his level. His power is so great, he broke through the floor at two venues we played.

—FROM "LOU REED: THE TAIJI RAVEN SPEAKS,"
BY MARTHA BURR, *KUNG FU TAI CHI* MAGAZINE, MAY/JUNE 2003

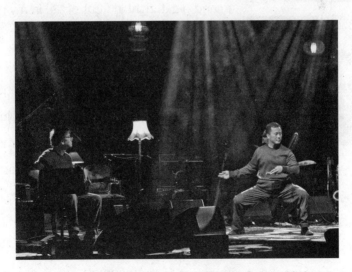

Lou and Ren onstage at the Vivid Festival, Sydney, 2010

I love martial arts people. I really do. I've only been really at two schools, but we have volunteer classes—guys get together and whatnot. I just think martial arts people are the greatest people. They always go out of their way. I haven't run into the archetype bad martial arts people that

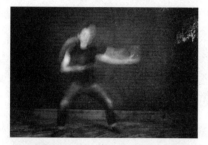

you hear about. . . . In our class, it's a "demographic" of people who normally probably wouldn't meet. It covers all spectrums so it really is interesting. A lot of musicians. . . .

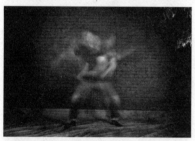

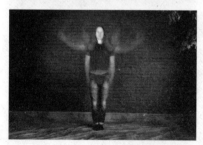

We took Master Ren on a world tour. We had a thing we did called "The Raven" where I was reading Edgar Allan Poe's "The Raven," that I'd rewritten. And we would have amorphous free-flow music. And Ren just stepped right in and did it, right in front of us. In my mind, I knew that he's so talented. I mean Chen Tai Chi as he does it is, amongst everything else, astonishing choreography. The difference between it and dance is the power, plus this marriage of doctors and fighters, merging

together so you could stay in shape, fight, and still have a rotator cuff at the end of the day. I don't know any other system where they were that smart to figure something like that out. That's amazing. Remember that documentary film with Samuel Jackson about martial arts [*The Art of Action: Martial Arts in the Movies*, 2002]? In there they said if you're looking at someone like Ren, you're looking at a Baryshnikov or a Nureyev. Now, ballet dancers can do those kicks, but it doesn't have the power. But Ren does. Given a choice of being kicked by one of the three, Ren wouldn't even be on the list. I wouldn't even think of it. His fajin, even if he doesn't touch you, the force zaps you. A lot of people talk about internal power, but you see it with Ren. . . .

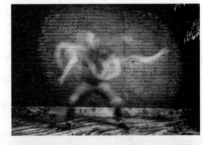

The "traditional" music has been tacked on from various sources. It's not even special music. Some of it's just a pop standard from Chinese radio in the '30s, as it turns out. It wasn't specially made by Cheng Man-ch'ing or something. It wasn't for Tai Chi. It just happened that way. I thought we could at least do as good as that. I had a lot of experience playing in back of Ren. . . .

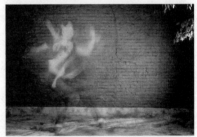

When Chen Xiaowang is around, he's always saying, "Calm down." In my older school, it was "Three deep breaths." They all have versions of it. So I said, "That's centering." And

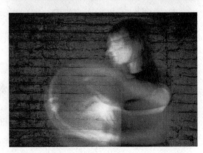

Lou's photos capturing the energy of Tai Chi

this means you can do that effect and not get thrown off, and the rhythm won't mess with you however you do it. The fast one, that's if you want to fly the plane. I do that. I just have so much fun doing that, it's amazing. Because it's real. It's not just there. It's actually doing something. It's really fun, really exciting. It couldn't be more opposite to what people are used to than if you sought out to do it on purpose, which we didn't. It was just to do something contemporary with it because I think Tai Chi is traditional but very, very contemporary. . . .

FlipperVision is seventeen, eighteen hundred photos that Martin von Haselberg took. If you stop that, it's not a form of video or freeze frame. This is an actual picture. And I said, "Hey, if you flip them, it moves just like those things you can buy. . . . We should put it in there just like that instead of a video that you pause." The thing is, "slideshow" exists all along, but this is a slideshow on steroids. Martin, a big-time martial arts fan and practitioner, took two thousand photos. Digital. Each file is like ten megabytes. And then they made a selection somehow, I can't even imagine, but anyway, they got it down to seventeen hundred or eighteen hundred. What else could you do with it? It's not a movie. It is the best educational thing I've ever seen because you can watch the video, but then you can watch him doing it. We were a little worried that you can't tell if he's moved here, there, or wherever—well, you're looking at that after you saw the video. What you're looking at is the alignment. This is where this is and it's within a fraction of a second. It's fantastic. . . . We sat there and said, "This should be released as a work of art. We should just stop right now. This thing is so beautiful." . . .

Indeed, crank up the volume of the energy music on the FlipperVision section, especially the straight sword, and art happens. This could play in the galleries of the Museum of Modern Art. In every shot, Ren is aligned.

It's just unbelievable. He's that good. I have been watching it and I've already corrected myself with so many little things. Because no one can tell you all of this stuff; it's impossible. . . .

And we thought this system, what it does aesthetically, physically, mentally, spiritually, in every way, this incredible life-enhancing force—not bad, right? [*laughs*]—should be seen. Yoga has had its time. Tae Bo, all of these things, great. . . . You have to know the form. Then you just get this energy out. It's really great. . . .

And there we are—this small gathering of students—we want Master Ren to reach more people with this. So we've been working very hard to try to make this happen. Yeah, there are other ones we're planning on—trying to keep that level of cinematography and sound. . . .

I'm putting out this meditation CD. It's three pieces of music. The second piece of music, it's fantastic for the same application—the Chen Tai Chi form—it's fantastic! But I made it for this meditation CD. At home, Ren heard it and said, "Hey! It's another one!" I said, "Can't we please have two uses for it?" and the answer so far has been "No." The record company said, "Please don't ask me to do this." Anyway, that's business. "A" doesn't want "B" to have it.

—FROM "LOU REED ON TAI CHI," BY
GENE CHING, *KUNG FU TAI CHI* MAGAZINE, JUNE 1, 2012

From an interview with Lou by Bob Belinoff, "Sitting Down with Lou Reed: On Tai Chi, Meditation Music, and Care of the Knees," LA Yoga *magazine, June 2007*

LOU REED: I had made *Hudson River Wind Meditations* for myself. Just for a number of different uses, and meditation, bodywork, Tai Chi, and I also would just leave it on all day . . . because it absorbs the outside sounds that might be irritating otherwise. It blends it into whatever's going on, for some reason. I don't know why that worked, but it did. So I just have it on all day, and it's just filling things in and making it nice. And I use it for the meditation. People started saying to me, "Can I have a copy of that?" you know, "Can you put that music on?" So I did that enough, and then after a while, I thought, *This is really great*, you know. We put just the music out on the theory that you probably have your own meditation you're doing and this is a great music to do it to rather than me putting the voice on it. . . .

BOB BELINOFF: The "Find Your Note" piece . . . there's the sound of a glass bowl almost.

LOU: Well, it could be a lot of things . . . but a glass bowl is good enough.

BOB: So you did this, essentially did this music for yourself?

LOU: I did it a hundred percent for myself.

BOB: And what kind of reaction have you gotten so far from it being out there?

LOU: People seem to respond to it in the spirit in which it was put out. I mean it is what it is. What I like about it is that it's not traditional and it's very modern and contemporary. And it has certain goals in mind; I think it accomplishes them.

BOB: I'm sure it does.

LOU: I'm not different from you or any other people. If it works for me, it works for you.

BOB: And the goal being . . .

LOU: To help you meditate. Or to work at anything where you know the music can be meditative or energizing depending on how you're listening to it. And, like I said, it can be an overall aural blanket.

BOB: Your music has always been for me, and I think for many people, part of an edge in the cultural milieu, it's been on the edge.

LOU: Well, there's no edge on this, although people would say me even putting it out is on the edge . . .

BOB: Yes, absolutely.

LOU: To my own career, I mean.

BOB: Well, that's true. Are you concerned with what people think?

LOU: If I ever listened to what other people think about anything . . . I would grind to a halt. I don't have any interest in that side of it or view of it at all.

BOB: That's never been a part of your craft?

LOU: Yep. Yep. I'm very hardcore. I follow the bouncing ball wherever it goes, and I don't care.

BOB: And when you first started to practice Tai Chi twenty years ago, twenty-five years ago . . . Did that change the kind of work you were doing in music, really, your approach to what you were creating?

LOU: Learning the fundamentals of foundational strength and alignment is a real big deal . . . and you can't lose for knowing that. I wish I'd been a little smarter then than I was, but it's taken a long time for me to realize the, you know, complexity and simplicity of what I've been taught and the ramifications it has on just things like walking and breathing, more or less doing something. And at that point I think I'd have to say goodbye because I have to get to the studio, okay?

From "Mass Destruction: Lou Reed and Stephan Berwick Talk Final Weapon,"
interview by Liz Belilovskaya, Planet III, April 2012

LIZ BELILOVSKAYA: How did you meet Ren? Correct me if I'm wrong but you've been doing Tai Chi for thirty years?

LOU REED: Yeah, but not his. He is a physical genius, a physical genius. The way he moves his body is beyond belief. He does it just in front of you, anyone, no matter what person it is, when they see him doing it, they sign up immediately. My point of view, if I can do one-thousandth of that thing, the day I saw that, I said to myself, "I am in the wrong part of town and I should have been over here." And then the word was that the class was so hard and that each step, each movement was controlled. So we just snuck in and started to get to know him and the other people there and enrolled.

LIZ: How long before you met Ren had you been doing the other types of Tai Chi?

LOU: Twenty to twenty-five years, uhh, twenty-five to twenty-seven years.

LIZ: When did you discover it initially and how?

LOU: I wanted a form of exercise that was useful. Not just cardio . . . I figured if I was going to do that, it should also be like self-defense and it should be beautiful, that led me to Eagle Claw, that led to Wu style, but it's nowhere near this.

[*Stephan and Lou met through Ren, they were his Tai Chi students. The three are now friends and collaborators.*]

LIZ: So, what I wanted to ask, the music that was selected for this film, talking to Stephan now—you selected the music? I thought Lou selected the music. So what I wanted to actually ask if any of the music selected—

LOU: I gave him access to certain things, and he looked at it and I said, yes, no, yes, no, or whatever.

LIZ: Are any of these selections from *Metal Machine Music*?

LOU: No.

STEPHAN BERWICK: No.

LIZ: Okay. The world tour for *NYC Man*, is this when you first realized that Ren could be a movie star? When he performed Tai Chi to your performances?

LOU: I always thought Master Ren was so exotic looking and so photogenic and because he's got such total control over his body, he could mimic and do practically anything, that he was made for movies.

LIZ: My question is why did you decide to use vintage music of Lou's instead of having him write something new?

LOU: First of all, I don't think of it as vintage.

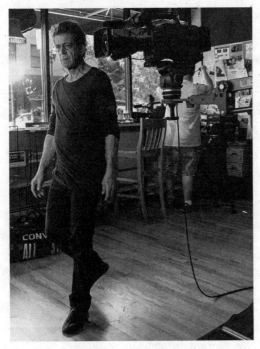

On the set of Final Weapon, *a short film directed by Stephan Berwick, 2010*

LIZ: That was the way it was described.

STEPHAN: Yeah, yeah.

LOU: I told you, I told you, I told you.

STEPHAN: I took down a lot of stuff. She must have—

LOU: I'm just saying, you see what I mean?

STEPHAN: I know what you mean. People immediately—

LOU: I think of it as timeless; it's an unfortunate choice of words by some people. With seven hundred songs, we could certainly find something that is responding to that kind of power because my music is about power.

STEPHAN: Yes.

LOU: So it was like a marriage made. All we had to do was find the ones that really did that.

LIZ: So the reason I ask is because I know that you have written music for some of Ren's instructional videos, right?

LOU: Yeah.

LIZ: So I was just kind of wondering why you chose not to do that for this film?

LOU: Because the other stuff does not have a drum, and a whole band in the back of it.

LIZ: I see.

LOU: You know, and this is analogue into digital and really has a real air and real drums.

STEPHAN: Something I really wanted.

LOU: And I wanted that power, I wanted that thing, when he brought it in to kick like Ren could kick, except musically.

LIZ: What is the most personal aspect of having this film made for you, is it just sharing your love of Tai Chi, is it about sharing its beauty?

LOU: It is a passion being presented to other people, trying to show them the beauty and the aesthetic value of all of this in twenty minutes and trying to use sound and picture to communicate this incredible aesthetic.

From Q&A with Lou, Stephan Berwick, Ren GuangYi, and co-founder and director Jonas Mekas after a screening of Final Weapon, *April 10, 2012, at Anthology Film Archives, New York, moderated by Scott Richman*

LOU REED: We heard that Ren's original class was a little rough.

SCOTT RICHMAN: What do you mean by a little rough?

LOU: You could really get hurt [*laughing*]. No protection, anyway, then he moved from Flushing, Queens, down to New York, and we went down to see him. He did some stuff and we said, "Oh my God . . . I've got to learn how to do one one-thousandth of that," and that was it, and I've been seeing him every day ever since. You see it in the movie. One of the things I think that's so great about the movie is that first you see him doing the form and it's like for once you get to really see it so beautiful, so powerful, and so matched to the music, and then he does this thing where he comes out of the house and the two guys jump on him and you feel the power. You know it's kind of all about power and you feel it. It comes right through for me, anyway. I don't know about other people. So I'm in love with it, always have been in love with it. Master Ren, if I could ever do a penny of that, I'd be a happy student. And I love the weapons forms, for instance. You know, kwan dao and the spear. Oh my, it's really great. Too bad we can't carry on the street.

SCOTT: Or through the airport.

LOU: I did, but they took them away.

SCOTT: So what do you use now when you go to the airport?

LOU: A gun. [*Audience laughs*.] You can have this, but the sky's the limit on the rest of it. See what you think, and that's what Stephan did, and he's got a real ear to match to video, because the music was about power. I think the movie is about power, and the music should really, really hit you when Ren hits you, and I just love that. That's where Stephan was placing things.

You know, there are all these beautiful pictures you can see if you read up on this a little bit, of one guy handing the other, you know, the Chen book of movements. It's incredible. That stuff is all real.

STEPHAN BERWICK: Yeah, it's all part of old Chinese martial arts. Some of it true, some not true, where things are codified, passed down in books tightly held just like a nuclear bomb. You know what I mean? It's tightly held by a few people who are given responsibility to use it and only a few people given responsibility to protect it.

TONY VISCONTI (from the audience): I got a quick question: We had a benefit a couple of years ago, and at the last minute Lou decided, which I thought was quite amazing to play, Maya Deren's *Meditation on Violence*, which is an amazing film featuring a Kung Fu master, and I was wondering what history Lou has with that film. I know that you truly appreciated Maya Deren before you chose it. I wondered what history you have with Deren's work and maybe that film as a martial art film, early experience.

LOU: I must've watched it a thousand times, so the idea of being able to put music to it was daunting and irresistible. She did that in, what,

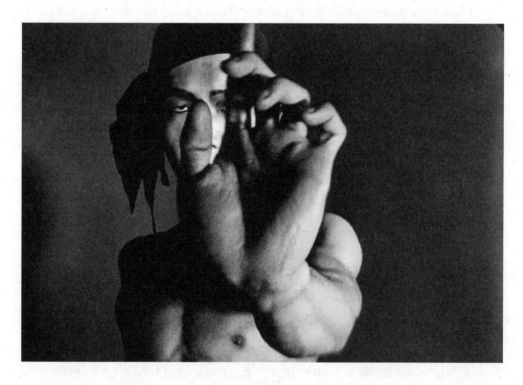

The American dance and film artist Maya Deren featured Yang-style Tai Chi and other Chinese martial arts in her 1948 film Meditation on Violence, *performed by the Chinese American actor and martial artist Chao-Li Chi*

[the] 1940s? Amazing, amazingly beautiful movie centered around this martial arts practitioner. I've watched it so often that I can't figure out, is he blind? You know, it's like he's in another state. In the photography, she's amazing. Imagine being that smart, that talented then, for an audience of, what, zero? It's kind of like liking good music now. [*Audience laughs.*]

SCOTT: The form Compact Cannon Fist was designed by Master Ren for Hugh Jackman to perform in the film *The Fountain*. The director, Darren Aronofsky, and his associate producer, Ari Handel, actually became aware of Master Ren. They looked him up and saw that he obviously had the skills as a great practitioner of Chen-style Tai Chi. When they got in touch with Ren, they explained the premise of the film to him, by which Master Ren then gave a demonstration. Both Darren and Ari were suitably convinced that he could then teach the principal lead in the film, Hugh Jackman, to do this form, Compact Cannon Fist. The form is featured prominently in the film. You taught Hugh Jackman for, I think, how many sessions? How many times did you teach Hugh Jackman?

REN GUANGYI: Yeah, three or four months. Every time I teach him was one hour. You know, for one hour at a time. Hugh Jackman was in a Broadway show seven days per week. That's a lot of work. He's very, very good. He's very, very nice. He's very pleasant. He's a very serious trainee. But always his stance is not very low in the beginning. A half year later, then things were very much better.

LOU: I was looking for this thing that actually would do exactly what it's doing. I was trying a lot of different ways to get there. I've had an interest in this for a really long time. Some of my interests in this are kind of infamous. I had in mind what I wanted, I just didn't quite know how to get there. I knew a lot of things not to do, but I didn't really have all the things that you should do. I know there's a lot of music out there that does this type of thing, or tries to do this type of thing. But that wasn't what I wanted to hear either. I wanted to hear exactly what you're hearing.

ANNE WALDMAN

Poet and founder/director, with Allen Ginsberg, of the Jack Kerouac School of Disembodied Poetics at Naropa University

I wrote several poems when Lou died, one that chants *Om Mani Padme Hum,* and I quote him in another with the title "New Scar Right Over My Heart." Which is how we were all feeling. And then again from Lou, "I fly right through this storm and I wake up in the calm" from "Magician (Internally)." This was consoling. His words, his poetry, always soaring, true. Also, his mentor Delmore Schwartz's line at hand: "It is the city consciousness, which sees and says: more: more and more: always more." When a poet dies, go to their poetry. And Lou carries the pulse for me of New York City, the vibratory liberated kinetics of such a maelstrom, such a history.

I feel so blessed, and every day I thank my generation for the amazing work that is, especially in these precarious times, life-sustaining. And I appreciate all the artists, seers, who've worked with meditative practices, showing the way, as Lou did.

Ancient wisdom practice such as Tai Chi has to do with synchronizing body, speech, and mind. Finding the jewels in the lotus. And the precision of the spiritual warrior.

So I'm feeling sustained by Lou's example. When we met in the 1960s this radical downtown art world was really explosive and coming together as a force. So, we overlapped in various ways. I met Lou pretty early on, and he gave me some poems that were in the book the Lou Reed Archive published *Do Angels Need Haircuts?* It was '71 when he was reading some of those early poems. I had known some of Delmore Schwartz's work, but now I look back and think, *My God. All these luminous coincidences and details of intergenerational intersection.* The sense of lineage, passing stuff on in the continuum in the ongoing rhizome.

We were all young. I mean this was like the start. It was great, but we weren't formed yet, kind of inchoate, and it was all happening, all the beautiful chaos, and love and drama, and collaborations. Transformative.

We started the St. Mark's Church Poetry Project in 1966. Lou showed up at events, gave the famous reading with Gerard Malanga. I was around the Factory a bit, was close to Gerard, John Giorno, and Rene Ricard. Ted Berrigan and I would stop in; we knew Andy, and Jackie Curtis. I lived at 33 St. Mark's Place, and was going regularly to the Velvet shows, and the whole scene; the poetry hub of St. Mark's and my apartment was generative. The gypsies lived below with stunning children and misty fortunes and the numbers racket. I was there for decades. It's now a tattoo parlor.

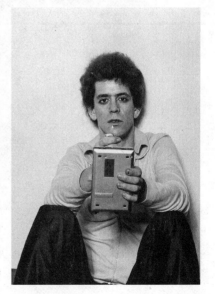

So I saw Lou most in the early days around the Velvets, and there was the scene, music and poetry and art and film. There were loft parties, openings, and shows. I went out to Boulder, to help found Naropa, '74; I got caught up in that vortex with its Buddhist backdrop and the lineages of the New American Poetry. What I call Outrider. Allen Ginsberg and I would sort of spell each other there. I had a child in 1980 and

Lou in the mid-'70s

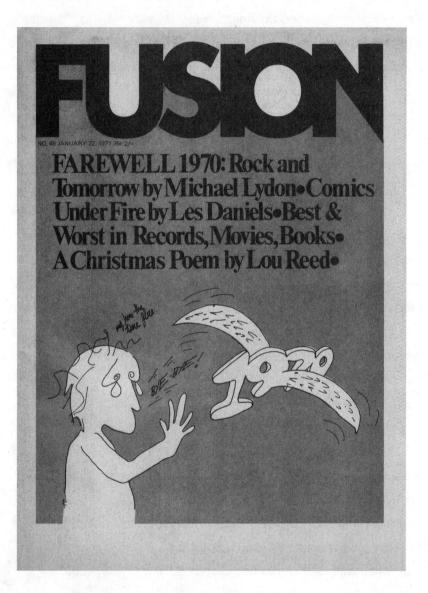

Fusion *48, 1971*

my center was Boulder for a while, although I was coming back and forth a lot. I would come into town, and I'd get into a concert, and would see Lou occasionally. Things grew in so many different ways, and also with the fame of somebody like Lou, you're going to the bigger venues.

SCOTT RICHMAN: What was Lou like in 1971?

ANNE WALDMAN: Curious. Open. Young. Gorgeous, mysterious. Very smart. Incredibly smart. A reader. Could be punk, contentious. Witty too. Didn't suffer fools. A poet. I thought of him as *poet* first of all. He talked about T. S. Eliot, "The Waste Land," William Burroughs.

SCOTT: And what was the reaction of the group when Lou went to rock 'n' roll?

ANNE: It was exciting, we followed him, but it took him on another trajectory. He was less accessible. I also like to get up and perform and sing and always thought you can do both—but I wasn't going to have a career of it, and there were geniuses like Lou who were full-on. He really went fully into it. We kind of lost him in that poetry community way, the way poets come and help collate and staple little mimeo magazines. He wasn't publishing tomes of poetry, but making brilliant records instead.

The Goddess Muse of rock comes and summons you. You have this huge platform and you're answering the call. A call of the performative imagination. Lou was an amazing performer; beautiful, heady, unpredictable. An original voice and distinctive sound, and sexy. And all these multiple shape-shifting personas and costumes, and different faces and moods. He's the non-binary trickster. The albums are complete worlds and works in and of themselves. Stories, epic poems. But he wasn't following the usual path of what a poet does. His study and mastery with Tai Chi was a steady path and he joined the sangha of practitioners and he became a "stream enterer," another artful form of life.

New Scar
Right Over My
Heart
by Anne Waldman

"We are the
insects of someone
else's thought."
—from "We Are the
People" by Lou Reed

takes the breath
away
steady raga
reticulated
sound downtown
sound
rounded and
turning and
pulse a subtle
strident
firing sound down
rebounded ritual
tone down
again . . . a round
again elfin effort
lou lou lou loop
  again
youth's pure-light
in maelstrom haze
of fabulous
below 14th Street
belletristic
atavistic time,
a world age,
radical, spiked
where you figure
it out,
cavalier
spin it out
instinct questions
narrative
branches of veins
work together
in a ritual form
tai chi will find
  life in

Andy, put your
teeth in us
  a catalyst
workaholic's
thrum
long DOM nights
just down the block
Mary Woronov
cracks
a whip
now better jump
through hoop of fire
work
in new light, Nico
part of allegory of
struggle we're in,
"the women in the
  room"
serial poem
walk into this room,
walk into
next room,
pulsing
never close
the door
into room beyond
room
inside room
fun house mirror
part of the *epikos*,
odyssey of body
time
ballade, rondeau
part of mystery
play,
or medieval tryst
an Elizabethan
drama
for your
Renaissance
thoughts
& attendant
sexy characters
flamed out or
  flaming within
re-constituted in
  transmigratory

void
a rock song, is ying
is yang?
many personae
approximate
tribulations and
deep loves of
Dante
you are T. S. Eliot's
fisher king
dented, distressed
grail of hope
how empty
is the cup,
how full a draught
warm elixir to
jester-oblivion
rock-poet, turn it
around
make magic
as free spirit
denizen
mystical way
out of hell
a left hand
path
gaping maw of the
hungry wasteland
ghost
realm
William Burroughs
  summons
you give
account of demons
or slink through
pale corridors
rock it in
crazy-wisdom
obstinate fun
power-sylphs
live in the
silky shadows
lust-realm and
anything you want
to possess, imbibe,
a sweet
lusting body

while seat gets hot
animal realm's
predatory drive
though the animals
will
smile at you—
something to tell
you
in samadhi,
come into
*our yelping theta
  zone . . .*
passionate under
  a sweeping
zeitgeist
gods war over your
  head
carnivalesque
backdrop's blood
evisceration
but hip to the street
broken vertebrae
of our century
  skips a beat
aches
how stretch
back in tendon
empathy,
get tough sullen
professional
obviate
  the cause, our
hands
are clean
or torqued
Lou you never say
  so
but go into it
into *form*
into *voice*
into *imago*
*the martial flying
warrior
sword strapped to
  back*
roll up sleeves
get all guitar-techy

science of the art is
imagination
what has also
come
down
panoramically
cool
"intellectual"
humanity's edge
  plays
loud decibels
kicks under
peoples' stories,
urban mix,
metabolic
  wry irony
underneath:
poetry's heart
everybody knows
someone
who is everybody's
other
story who is
some other one's
fool
  emotion
everybody says
as Candy says
knows everybody
who
  is everybody's
squeeze
one's connection
one's bliss
and now what
are we inside
crux of,
my man,
*white veins running
through cheeks*
what sky gazing at
waits at desire
on the neuron path
where light
hasn't reached us
but already
happened

anticipates a
future
without you & with
you
asides, cracks
generative
darkness as
cells churn
pale eye retina
gleams then blurs
vocals
create
ontogeny, a voice
more blue
counter-
revolutionary
civilians
in a voice? did
voice
own it? the time?
our own Kulchur
with a capital "K"?
how lucky
you are
New York we
  invented you
create you in
our wild image
get down and listen
don't just
weep the gone
times
remember through
meme loops
a native son
his streets
lou lou lou lou
  loosens
  his mortal loop,
meets death in love
with softness
tai chi—the
boundless first
part of
survival's trickster
Masquerade.

HAL WILLNER

Producer and curator for music, film, TV, and theater; creator of the TV series Night Music; *co-host of the radio show* New York Shuffle; *and Lou's best friend*

I met Lou in 1985. Things were beginning to change. Before that he was probably very cuckoo. It was an amazing period.

He taught me to be a producer. Part of the Stravinsky definition of one is to listen, have a good sense of the history of music, be a child psychiatrist and a liar. Lou made me a producer.

With Lou, you saw an artist always in transition, never standing still, always looking for the next part. Taking risks and knowing it's about great poets and writers and artists, and knowing there are going to be hills and valleys. Maybe it's not accepting the valleys as valleys.

He never repeated himself. Every time he made a record that crossed over into the mainstream, he always followed it, and not purposely, with a record that would almost ruin his career. *Transformer* was followed by

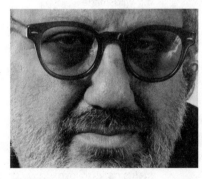

Berlin. I believe *Sally Can't Dance* was followed by *Metal Machine Music*, and *New York* was followed by *Magic and Loss*. It's amazing. He started to look at it humorously. I'll never forget his impression of Seymour Stein when he hands him *Magic and Loss* after the huge hit of *New York* and "Dirty Blvd." He imitated him like Curly from the Three Stooges, "What are you giving me here? There's no songs about kids? I mean come on."

Hal Willner

You are looking at an artist who doesn't rest on his laurels, and doesn't become another Vegas act like so many others. Thinking of Vegas, how about when he played there at the Hard Rock and wouldn't play until they shut down the slots. I mean taking on the mafia. They turned them off. Who does that?

You can see that Tai Chi was part of his development. Listen to the difference between "Sister Ray" and "Like a Possum." They have a similar mindset, but one is meditative and one is angry. "Like a Possum" is not angry. It's humor. It's meditative.

Tai Chi was backing Lou's music in a hypnotic way.

Tai Chi was backing Lou's music in a hypnotic way without seeing it. When most of us in this country saw it for the first time, Tai Chi was a total cartoon. It was all about hurting someone, about defending, and nothing else, except maybe for *Kung Fu*, David Carradine's show. That's what it was. That's what we learned about.

There is more. There's the spiritual part of it, what it meant for your mind.

How does someone clear their mind? For me, jumping in the ocean

▲

does that. Some other people, it's golf. It's Tai Chi that kept Lou alive. He would have left us much earlier if it wasn't for that. I mean you can tell it realigned his organs and his mental state.

Being on tour, everyone becomes road weary on the bus, except Master Ren. He was amazing. I understand that Tai Chi became a part of Lou's art and so did Ren. We were do-ing an evening of Edgar Allan Poe at Royce Hall UCLA. It was really stressful. It was crazy important that Ren was there—just his right arm, really. It was important to him so it was im-portant to us. We worked closely, really closely over the last ten years of Lou's life, so I saw the change. You could see how much more impor-tant it became to him.

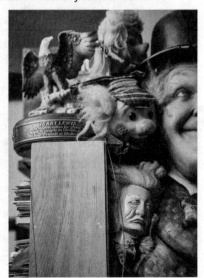

Puppets were everywhere in Willner's Midtown studio

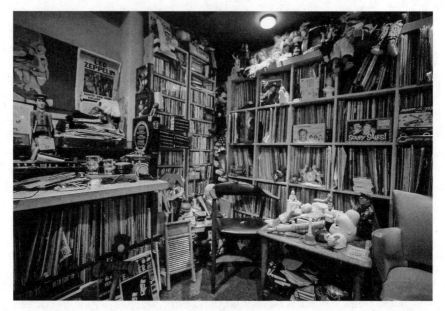

Willner's studio: an eclectic and encyclopedic mix of many eras of music and television

He tried to get others interested. Tony. Fernando. I don't think Tony went for it, though I heard he tried it. People just saw how it kept Lou alive. I mean Lou wasn't pushing a cult conversion.

I'm sure I've had some martial arts people. No one comes to mind. Allen Ginsberg practiced Tai Chi. I know that Burroughs was the opposite of Allen. He was very cynical about the whole thing, but he'd just say, "Ah, come on. Hey, Marcel Marceau, look at this shit." That's what it reminded him of. But that's what made that stuff work. He had no patience.

But I had to do it my own way. I'm not going into a hot, sweaty room. I can't deal with that. But with meditation I totally got it.

Let's just say, a lot of us had our dangerous period of substance abuse and whatever that was. I did, and Lou did a lot to bring down my addiction. It was a very hard thing. So meditation is something I learned in coming out of that. Allen Ginsberg taught me this. I learned music is breath. It really is breath. I related to that easily. But Lou couldn't have been more supportive. It wasn't easy to kick after twenty-five of my forty years.

It took me a year and a half to pull out of it, and Lou simply said, "You know, I can't really trust you right now with this," so we didn't speak for a year. If I saw him, he wouldn't look at me, and then I guess he heard or felt something. Fernando called and said, "Lou's been asking about you." I saw him then in 1998 at the Knitting Factory. Lou just had that smile. He could tell. He could tell right off. And then a huge hug, a great one. He came over the next day, we sat, and he started with, "I don't like many people, but I like you."

In 2008, we started doing a radio show on Sirius Radio, *New York Shuffle*, out of Lou's apartment. We did it there, rather than a studio, be- *I learned* cause the magic of those shows was, we forgot we were doing a radio *music* show. For half of the show, we played music that we loved, and the other *is breath.* half was music we hadn't heard before. We built the show with the idea it was against the record business philosophy of two great songs and the ▲ rest filler. No artist we have any respect for puts filler on their record. So we'd get a new album by an artist and hit shuffle, play whatever came up. It was discovery for us. Chasing obsessions.

Tai Chi shows up here too because of what it does to the brain. I'm sure it affects emotion. He would show his goose bumps or break into tears when he heard or saw something beautiful. He could get right to the heart of the music, and he was very hurt if you didn't try. I pestered him once about the music at Levon Helm's Midnight Ramble when he came back after seeing it upstate. What it was like and all that. He finally said, "What do you want me to tell you? It's good-time music. It's like your puppy dog." He understood rock and roll was often good-time music, but it could be so much more. He wanted to bring in the influences of Delmore Schwartz and all that stuff.

He always made work about what he was going through. The angry period. The happy period. Lou was in excruciating pain while making *Lulu*, his last record. If you listen, it's interesting; Warren Zevon's last record, or Leonard Cohen's, even Bowie's, it's "Ready, my Lord." Lou was not "Ready, my Lord." He was "Fuck you, Lord!" It was a fuck-you record. David Bowie pointed out it might be the most honest record ever.

JULIAN SCHNABEL

Friend, artist, and film director; director of Berlin

I knew Lou's music before I knew Lou. *Berlin*—I think it came out in 1973—made a huge impression on me, and I listened to it for about five years. All the time. I was in Germany in 1978, installing a show, the first show I had

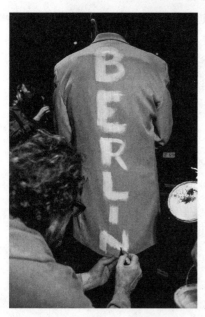

in Europe, and I was still listening to the record. And I guess I'd imagined that he actually was in Berlin and all this happened there. Later I found out that it really all happened in New York, but that didn't really matter because my experience in Germany was colored by his imagination.

I met Lou around 1987—the year Andy Warhol died—and I had this idea that we should make a requiem for Andy. I talked to John Cale about it at Andy's wake. I guess he spoke to Lou about doing it, and he told me Lou didn't want me to get involved because he thought I'd take over. And I said, "Why don't you guys just do it?"

I told Lou what happened, and he said that was absolutely ridiculous and that that

Bob Ezrin wore a jacket painted by Julian Schnabel for the Berlin *performances, Brooklyn, 2006*

didn't happen at all. From that moment on we became great friends—as if we grew up together. And we did all sorts of things together. We had a great love. I had a great love for him, and I always felt like I got the ball back in my court right away, and maybe he felt like that too. Now I live across the street, and I would see Lou on the roof with Master Ren, practicing. I really enjoyed watching them. And now that I've rebuilt my own building and they could look over there at me too.

And I just knew how much it meant to Lou, because I feel like when he did that, it kind of took him to this other place, an otherworldly place where I feel like his spirit and his soul revived. I think Lou wanted Master Ren to go with him when he went on concert tours because Master Ren had an energy that regenerated Lou and made him feel powerful.

I think Lou tried to make a portrait of Tai Chi through music, of the feeling he got from this practice. I think it's very hard to do and maybe this is why you're making a book. I don't know. It seems very hard to describe what that thing is. It was almost as if he made a painting when he made the music for Master Ren. He had this incredible respect and love for this man, which was quite infectious. Everybody who was important to Lou met Master Ren and had to think about this man seriously, and it wasn't for nothing either.

If I remember correctly, the day after Lou died, we were all out in the sand dunes, and everyone who took this walk into the sand dunes practiced Tai Chi that day. Somehow in the movement of the air and being in that place all together, I think that we all had some kind of a communal wave that ran through us. It was an incredible bond. I think we felt Lou coming through us as that was happening. I think it was extremely comforting to him. And it was comforting to the people who were doing it on the dunes. It's probably very comforting to you too, Laurie. You can connect with him when you're doing it. Maybe I feel a little lazier. Sometimes it's almost like we're too busy to do things that are really important. So I haven't been involved in practicing it, but I certainly can feel how meaningful it was to him and to you.

LAURIE ANDERSON: How did you feel about Lou trying to bring Tai Chi to a wider audience?

JULIAN SCHNABEL: Well, in a sense, it's like trying to put a square block in a round hole, because people are not necessarily ready to make that leap. But that being said, it never stopped Lou from trying to show people another way to look at things. And if you have witnessed Ren or have been close to him, or witnessed him up close and seen the kind of power and energy and control that must come from being connected to the center of something, that's something that is possible but very unusual for a human to do. There's a generosity and a profound connection with something that started a long time ago, maybe before thought. And I guess that was very attractive to Lou. And not in a glib sense. It seemed like kind of a shining light, and I think he tried to share that with other people.

It was electric. Lou was interested in electric music, and he was interested in electricity and the transferal of energy from one person to the next and what could be achieved with that. And I think absolutely the Tai Chi music was certainly part of the same suite of feeling and intention that took place in his last work, *Lulu*, which I think is a great psychedelic, a masterwork, really.

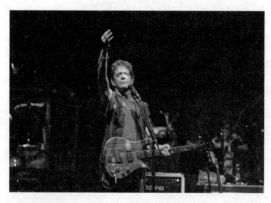
Berlin *on tour*

I don't know how many people do this, but I always like to think leaning towards a divine light is the way to go.

And I think that's what Lou was doing. And a light hit him, and I think that we're always trying to capture that energy. And somehow by recording this intention, there is a physical body in the music that permeates the air. Lou was hoping this body would be synonymous with this sensation.

Lou was interested in electric music, and he was interested in electricity and the transferal of energy from one person to the next.

▲

LAURIE: You made *Berlin*, the concert film, in 2007 that brought that record back to life. The three of us looked at the film the day before Lou died, and he spent the entire film laughing. He loved that film so much. Can you talk a little bit about working with him on that movie?

JULIAN: I remember when Lou first talked to me about the film. Initially he asked me if I would do the sets, and I said to him that "Well, they only have sixteen thousand dollars. We can't even get them over there for that. So I don't know how I'm supposed to make the art for this production. But why don't we do it a different way and you and me will pay for it? We'll put in fifty thousand dollars apiece and we'll film it and we'll own it, whatever it is? And we won't ask anybody for anything." You know, God bless the child that's got his own.

So we did that and then later we never made any money with it, but we got an immense amount of joy out of making this together and for me to watch Lou play that after thirty-five years and to watch him watching Steve Hunter and the different players playing was an amazing thing. When we were watching the movie that day at your house, he all of a sudden screamed at the TV, "Who paid for this? The authors!" And he forgot that he was dying.

Some things take you outside your limits, as your body is falling apart or whatever's happening, and you can be there. That's how you feel when you're making the art, and that's how you can feel if you're not the author of that work, just experiencing it, and that's maybe one of the reasons why people do it.

LAURIE: I was just thinking you probably had the most physical relationship with Lou other than Master Ren. That's just coming off the top of my head right now, because I'm just realizing how comfortable he felt with you.

JULIAN: The thing is that we spent a lot of time together. We lived across the street from each other, and when you were traveling, working, or performing somewhere, he missed you a lot. And he needed you a lot, and I guess I was the surrogate somehow.

I couldn't do all the same things that you do, but I could talk to him about a lot of things and listen to him and made no judgments about things, and I think he felt like we really grew up together and he could talk to me about anything. And I could talk to him about anything. When my father died, I asked Lou to come over, and the two of us sat there and looked at my father lying in the bed dead and he sat there with me.

SCOTT RICHMAN: You worked with Lou on *The Raven* years ago in 2001 and you did the photo shoot. How did that come about?

JULIAN: Well, I was out in Montauk, and I had this twenty-four-by-twenty-inch camera, and I had this old coat, and I had a couple of different things. I had an old car, and he came out with a sword. He liked swords. He liked swords and weapons. There was this old hat and this old coat there and a sword, and I felt like he looked like a world-weary samurai walking around there. Like he stepped out of a Tarkovsky movie. Or out of an Andrei Rublev or something.

But you know what it is? It's trust. I don't know how many people he trusted, but he did trust me, and I think when you work together and somebody trusts you, that's the basis of it. They'll let you do something because they want to see what you're going to do and they don't feel like

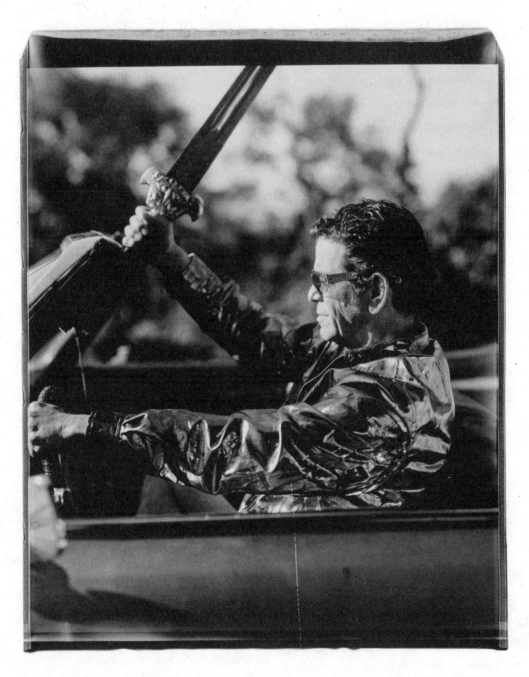

Portrait of Lou by Julian Schnabel used as the back cover image for The Raven *album, 2003*

you're going to rob them, steal something, or hurt what their impulse is. And so together we were able to make a lot of things that I think we both loved and enjoyed doing.

I feel really blessed to know him and also to know Laurie and actually really know profoundly how much they respected and cared for each other. I just feel lucky, because it's so terrifying to be alive, that I knew him and that I know her, because it's scary out there.

ROBERT WILSON

Creator and director of musical theater and opera, visual artist, and founder of the Watermill Center for the Arts

I first met Lou very briefly in the late '60s with Andy Warhol. I knew some people that knew Andy, and I had just gotten to know Fred Hughes, and I met Lou at Andy's Factory space. I saw him on occasion in the '70s, but I didn't really know him.

I begin to work by drawing. When I worked with Lou, I would make a sketch or a drawing and then Lou and I would talk about the nature of a scene. Should it be slow or quick or loud or quiet, and we worked very freely.

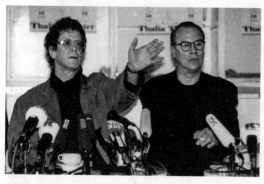

A press conference with Robert Wilson for their musical Time Rocker

I sketched a lot of the pieces we did together with existing music of his. Sometimes I would take an upbeat rock song and then I would slow it down. It was a real collaboration, a great dialogue, and it was easy for us to work. He said on different occasions that it was the same way that he worked with Andy and that in some ways I reminded him of Andy. As I said, sketches and drawings were how we always worked. Lou wasn't always there, especially for some of the rehearsals, so I would just sketch out the piece. The wonderful thing about Lou was he would provide me with a lot of music and sketches and tape, and he said, "You can place them the way you want."

I learned from him an appreciation for the loudness of a sound, and that space that is created with the loudness.

▲

Lou said he felt a closeness to my work because of an interest in Tai Chi. And I saw him on different occasions practicing Tai Chi. Actually, I never did study Tai Chi, but I felt an affinity with it because I had been very much influenced by the choreographer Suzushi Hanayagi. Her family goes back to the fourteenth century. It's the oldest living family of Japanese choreographers. Suzushi was trained in the Noh, Bunraku, and the Kabuki. She was a Noh actress, but at that time it was next to impossible for a woman to perform in the Noh theater because all the performers were men. Suzushi was trained from a very early age to do male parts, which were very close to martial arts. So Lou and I had this connection as well. When I met Suzushi in the late '70s and early '80s, my whole viewpoint of theater was reconfirmed by seeing her work. Suzushi later became a Zen Buddhist. She did very calm and meditative works that were contemporary choreography. What I admired most was her background and her training as a classical actor, especially in the Noh doing male roles. In the late '90s, she performed a male role at the National Theatre in Tokyo and that was quite an event. I saw her do that, and this was a kind of a connection that Lou and I had.

One additional thing I wanted to say about Lou was I learned from him an appreciation for the loudness of a sound, and that space that is created with the loudness. The beginning of *Time Rocker* with the steel guitar was so incredible. Some of the last music he wrote for *Lulu* was really about loudness. But on the other side, we shared a common aesthetic. He understood something very quiet and the softness of a sound. Some of the last music he did, like the song "Little Dog" and some of the music for *Lulu*, were very quiet and soft sounds, like the way snow can touch a peach and the way the sound then touches your ear. It's so amazing as an artist that he had this range and this vocabulary. He was a real friend, a great artist, and unequaled.

SARTH CALHOUN

Fellow student and electronic musician in Lou Reed's band

One day in about 1999, I saw a guy right at sunrise doing Chen Tai Chi in the Key Food parking lot near my house. I thought, *One day I'm going to do that. One day I will find a teacher.* And then a little bit later, I was asking my friend about Tai Chi and Chen style, and she recommended Master Ren. Said he was the best, so I came to his class.

We would usually start off with some standing meditation, then we would do Silk Reeling. And then we would take a short break and do a little bit of sort of goofing off and Push Hands and stuff. And then we would do the forms and then, after we went through the various different forms, we would again do some applications or Push Hands at the end of the class, and that's when it would get really kind of raucous.

SILK REELING describes the spooling movement of chi throughout the body. Chen Tai Chi's Silk Reeling training removes obstructions from the body's chi pathways to fortify the circulation of internal energy.

Lou was very into the martial aspects and also very opinionated about it. He would often give opinions about what I was doing when I was doing the Push Hands. Was it really Tai Chi? Was it using too much force? How was my technique? It was always a great topic of discussion and discovery.

Lou knew a lot about martial arts and had a lot of different perspectives from various things he studied. And he took the various teachings and information that he got from different people very seriously. He was really great to talk with about all these topics. He could analyze and dig deeper and sort of plan what each of us would work on next.

I've always been very interested in applications. Lou was obviously very interested in applications too. Many of us were. I feel that Master Ren did a really great job of showing how the applications are more principle based. So when you have a certain move for a form, there's not just one application for that. There are many different ways that movement can be used. Ren spent a lot of time to not think narrowly but to think about all the ways we could use the movements.

It's cultivating power and focusing power.

▲

I started to think about how music could maybe cause altered states in the same way a Tai Chi practice or a meditation practice. And maybe that was part of why I was drawn to Tai Chi. One of the weirdest things that happened when I first started doing Tai Chi was my hand independence on keyboards dramatically increased. So there's definitely some sort of relationship between musical instruments and Tai Chi, even if it's hard to pinpoint. It has something to do with the internal rhythm of the body. One of the interesting things about Chen style is that there's a very clear pace and phrasing to it. And I think there's a really intense sense of musicality there. I think that Lou's approach to Tai Chi was very musical and lyrical.

One of the things that was fun about Lou as an artist was how much he emphasized making abrupt changes during shows. You can get really loud right now or really quiet or totally change it. Chen is a great art in that way too. We can do these beautiful slow things and then just explode with power. Often when I talked with Lou about Tai Chi he would use the word "power." *Power*. And a lot of people don't use the word "power" when they talk about Tai Chi. For Lou and Master Ren, it's not only about grace or fluidity or fixing your knee. It's not only about calming your mind. It's cultivating power and focusing power.

I don't want to speak about Lou's deeper motivation because I feel I can never know why someone's doing something. What we talked about so enthusiastically was the martial aspect. We would often sort of laud the health benefits, like, oh, this is so great. It fixes your energy, it fixes your blood sugar, it makes you sleep better, you make your girlfriend happier. You would love to list all those things, but they're more, like, given. What was exciting and drove the pursuit was the martial aspect, the power.

Hudson River Wind Meditations is a really good purist template for the way music can represent the pulsing movement of Tai Chi. Tai Chi has a shift, turn, sink, shift, turn, sink, shift, turn, sink. Everything in the Chen style follows that pattern more or less, right? Shift, turn, sink, shift, turn, sink. It's like a wave. It never stops. It has moments of punctuation, but the underlying thing never stops. When we started making other pieces, they made us feel like we were doing Tai Chi. We had pieces for Cannon Fist, for the 21 Form. We had a piece for the 19 Form, and for Silk Reeling.

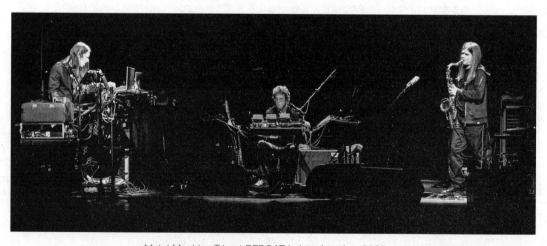

Metal Machine Trio at REDCAT in Los Angeles, 2008

Lou had this new camera and he brought that out and we bought some lights and stuff and really started to delve into this idea of doing a slideshow of the long exposures. All of a sudden, all of these shapes that people talk about in Tai Chi became obvious. Figure eights, spirals. It's very hard to see that otherwise.

On tour we would have the aspiration to practice every morning, but that wouldn't necessarily happen. Touring is difficult. We would try; we would often do a few minutes before we went out onstage.

Lou had a very specific way that he liked to practice. He liked to do the 19, 21, 38 Forms in sequence. That was his routine. But if we were doing it at the venue before we went onstage, we would do a little Silk Reeling and then 21 Form.

Tai Chi made me feel more committed to the idea that I want to create work that helps people reach a mental state that is healing or powerful and helps them change or alter themselves. In other words, the idea of music is to alter the listener's mental state and to be conscious of the way it's being altered. I've been doing work now that is basically Tai Chi meditation in music. I make drones and play Continuum keyboard melodies over them. The goal is to help people get into a meditative state.

ULRICH KRIEGER

Composer, saxophonist with Metal Machine Trio, and musician in Lou's touring band

We talked a lot about our individual approaches to feedback. I think we even talked about Edgard Varèse and his definition of music as organized sound. For me, *Metal Machine Music* is at the same time the ultimate rock and roll piece and a guitar version of an orchestral piece. And all of those elements of contemporary art music are in there. Maybe one of the first pieces to bring rock music into that world of art music.

I think that there's a clear link between *Metal Machine Music*, the Metal Machine Trio music, and Tai Chi. I really think the listening and the playing of that music takes a similar mindset.

I spoke with Lou about *Hudson River Wind Meditations* as being kind of a *Metal Machine Music*–related piece. Although it's much calmer, it's also much quieter. But I think we both agreed that *Hudson River Wind Meditations* definitely has strong ties to *Metal Machine Music* in the way, again, you listen and experience it.

RALPH GIBSON

Friend, photographer, collaborator on Red Shirley

Annie Ohayon introduced me to Lou, about fifteen years ago at a party at her house, and I guess it was what you call love at first sight. We certainly did click, and Lou said to me, "Call me for lunch anytime you want. I can go anytime—I'm self-employed." So we started having our lunches at Sant Ambroeus in the West Village. He loved photography, and our friendship grew.

He wanted me to be the cinematographer on the *Red Shirley* project, and I said no. I had done some documentary camerawork as a young man when the cameras were heavier, and I just didn't want to do it. He said, "Come over. I'll show you a tiny little camera." It was a Canon 5D digital. It's very important I point out, he kicked open the door of prejudice, which I had reinforced against digital. I just didn't want anything to do with it. But then I started fooling around with that little camera and saw that it had tremendous potential. I agreed to be the camera partner and collaborate with him on *Red Shirley*. This was a documentary about Lou's cousin Shirley.

In tennis, you exhale at the moment of impact. I exhale at the moment of releasing the shutter.

▲

All I did was, as a photographer, quickly recognize the incredible, tangible love between Shirley and Lou. All I had to do in terms of content was get it in focus. Then of course he was very aleatory in any style. He considered it a fifty-fifty collaboration. You know, Shirley emanated such a presence that she altered my sense of self as well as Lou's. I never saw him fawn like that over anyone. It was a genuine thing.

I never tried Tai Chi, but I recall a dinner when we spoke about his relationship to martial arts, Tai Chi, and photography. I had studied boxing for a few years, and I took a lot of lessons and sparred. I learned that it's very easy not to get hit if you know how to avoid it, and it's very hard to hit somebody who knows how not to get hit. But there is the shared information that is called "weight transfer." Lou and I talked about this.

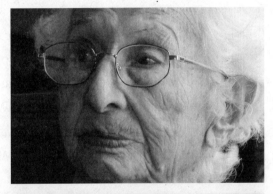

In tennis, you exhale at the moment of impact. I exhale at the moment of releasing the shutter, which he liked and totally grasped because of his Tai Chi practice, and I went on to say, you know, McEnroe could volley while he was backing up, exhaling, Muhammad Ali could jab while he was backing up, and Baryshnikov told me once that after thirty-two pirouettes at the peak of his arc he would exhale in midair, and the audience would gasp because he appeared to stop in midair.

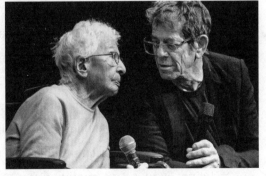

Above: Lou's cousin Shulamit Rabinowitz aka "Red Shirley"; below: Shulamit Rabinowitz and Lou Reed at the 20th Annual New York Jewish Film Festival premiere of Red Shirley *in New York City, 2011*

DARREN ARONOFSKY

Film director

Lou is from Brooklyn, I'm from Brooklyn and a lifelong New Yorker, and Lou is definitely the key poet of New York City. He was this legend that shone over most of the arts in New York. Lou was a huge fan of the writer Hubert Selby Jr. When I started to work on *Requiem for a Dream*, I went to Lou to talk about the possibility of him doing the music. If I'm right, that was his favorite Selby book. But Lou just didn't feel like he was a film composer. That wasn't his art. After that, I would see him now and then and hang out.

My memory of doing the Metallica video with him is just so rich. That was a real collaboration. We got to spend a couple of days together and really worked together on that. He was very complimentary of that work.

How this came about was I saw him at a dinner and he said, "Me and my band made an album and I want you to do the first video." I said, "Wow. That's amazing. I'd love to. Who's the band?" Because I didn't know he had a band. "Oh, Metallica."

He was always very supportive of me. He was very much a godfather to me. Whenever he would see me, he'd treat me very much like a son. He was just very warm. It's funny because he had a reputation for not being so warm and I never witnessed that ever. It was just pure warmth I felt from Lou.

I called up my producer and my cinematographer. "Lou Reed wants us to do a video with him and Metallica." We had a very limited budget. We shot it at Metallica's studio and went very lo-fi, back to black-and-white, like I did on my first films. Very, very grainy, very high contrast, and just worked with what we had. We built a black box and lit Lou and the band members in it. I was looking around for places to shoot and found these really distorted storm windows and we used them to create some warped images. There were no digital effects. It was basically using these shitty storm windows that had been there for twenty years and shaking them.

When we were shooting "The View," Lou started to cry. You look at the video, he's actually weeping. I don't know what it was about. I think it was the material was getting to him and it was a pretty intense moment to be a part of.

I wrote Tai Chi into *The Fountain*, and when it came time to actually make the movie, we needed to find a teacher for Hugh Jackman. I found Master Ren, and he was working with Lou. The thing I remember about working with Master Ren was, when he started to train Hugh, he went over to Hugh's house, and as he was demonstrating one of his kata—I'm not sure if that's what you call them—but he put his foot through Hugh's new floor. We all laughed and it was funny, and Hugh of course was a gentleman about it. Then, a few weeks later, he did it again. That's how much power he had.

I think the only time, though, I saw Lou do Tai Chi was when I went to a class to meet Master Ren. I went with Lou and to observe the class. Master Ren was teaching. I didn't know Master Ren, but in the end, everything reversed and he was auditioning me. I've done a little Tai Chi. Myself, I've been interested in the martial arts since I was a teenager. I've done a lot of different martial arts, and I did Tai Chi for a while. The way Lou was attracted to Tai Chi, I think he leaned on it to help him in so many different ways—it was an inspiration.

One last thing: I'm from Coney Island, so I've been going to the Mermaid Parade since back when there were more people in the parade than watching the parade. One year Lou and Laurie were king and queen.

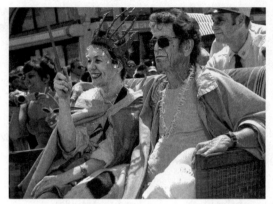

Laurie and Lou, King and Queen of the Coney Island Mermaid Parade, 2010

Lolabelle was there. We had the parade, then we went down to open up the beach. It's this great moment, and I remember Laurie and Lou wading into the ocean and everyone just dancing in the water. Great party. Great to have them there. They definitely were the best king and queen Coney Island ever had.

LARS ULRICH

Drummer, founding member of Metallica, and Lou's neighbor in New York City

The first time I met Lou was at Tivoli, the amusement park in Copenhagen, but our musical trajectory really started with the twenty-fifth anniversary celebration for the Rock and Roll Hall of Fame in 2009. We were to play with Ozzy Osbourne, Ray Davies, and Lou.

The show was in Madison Square Garden, and we came a few days early to rehearse. Lou came in and was ready, but he was a little unsure, trying to find a place in all our equipment and people. But once we started playing, any awkwardness disappeared and we fell into the music. We became very comfortable and in a couple of hours figured out what to do.

It was interesting. When we first met, Lou was very guarded. He kept people at bay. He wanted to know what people's motives were. But in a couple of hours, he went from guarded to a remarkable energy. From then on there was a closeness and trust. There was comfort in the strength of the group, and Lou figured out how to fit in.

In the bowels of Madison Square Garden, after the show, Lou said, "Let's make a record. Let's work on a project together one day." Those were his parting words, and a year or so later we picked it up. Lou said, "I'm gonna send you the lyrics and I want you and James [Hetfield] to start familiarizing yourself with the lyrics and start being inspired by the lyrics." We were completely game for this. We had a chance to get to a creative place we'd never been, and the lyrics inspired that. Lou took us out of our comfort zone.

The lyrics were angry, spiteful, awkward, and beautiful, and all made sense. It was a cohesive work that had almost every human emotion.

When *Lulu* was released, there was intensity in how people reacted. A negative one. What the fuck is it about *Lulu* that it got that kind of re-action? I can't quite figure it out, but years later, it's aged extremely well. It sounds like a motherfucker still. So I can only put the reaction down to ignorance. It brings out all kinds of emotions, and everyone is now a critic with a keyboard at their fingertips. It took our fans to a place I wish they would go more often. Maybe it would be a better time to release it now with what's going on outside in the world, the chaos. I don't know, but I am very proud of this record. The music and everything that came out of this collaboration was so precious and so alive. It was all created in these flashes of impulsive energy, and all these things just happened. James and I would be figuring out ways through a piece of music and then Lou would look over and go, "That's it. I'm not doing another fucking take of that." It's not the way we usually worked, but it was so beautiful and great, the whole thing.

It was all created in these flashes of impulsive energy.

▲

While making the record, Lou would go into the large space we had outside our studio in Marin and practice Tai Chi. I never was fully immersed in it with him. Like with his guitar setup, I tried my best to stay out of the

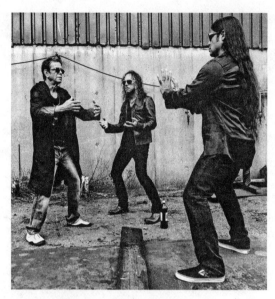
Lou practicing Tai Chi with Metallica

way. Kirk Hammett, our guitarist, is an avid Yoga practitioner, and the two of them connected.

Tai Chi was not at the very top of what Lou and I shared, but he would often talk about the discipline of it and the meditative state that would accompany it and so on, and I felt that it was a window into his personality. The one thing that was so beautiful about him, he never tried to apologize or excuse all the different things that lived inside him. I don't think I've ever met a person that was so unapologetic for what he was saying and how he was. He was just true to the moment and true to the mood and how he's feeling at the time. These games that we play, there was just nothing of that with Lou. And it was such a rare thing and such a beautiful thing to see somebody that was so comfortable with letting it all out there to be dissected for the masses. Tai Chi was a part of that, and I think it all fits together very well.

KIRK HAMMETT

Guitarist with Metallica and Yoga practitioner

Lou taught me how to be in the moment and trust my instincts as an artist. We weren't used to working that way in Metallica. And Lou taught me how to do that—and on *Lulu,* this last record, I would say nearly 90 percent of what I did on guitar was done that way. In the past, I would have worked something out for three months before getting into the studio. It changed the way I approached my work.

Lou used to go off in the middle of the day when we were in the studio, and we didn't know where he went. I went out one day to get some air and to meditate, and I found Lou outside doing his moves and forms with a sword. When you think of Lou, you don't think of Fred Astaire or someone. But he was so graceful.

JOSÉ FIGUEROA

Top-ranked Tai Chi competitor and first-generation student of Ren GuangYi

Before I practiced martial arts, I was break dancing. I was a part of the early hip-hop movement as a founding member of the Rock Steady Crew, with the group's co-founder, Jojo. We were actually watching Kung Fu films at the time, and a lot of what we came up with as break dancing were things we found in those movies. This is something that stuck with me for many years. I then searched for and learned different martial arts.

Tai Chi really did it for me. I started with Yang style, under Derrick Trent. In '91, I heard about a master from China in New York: Ren GuangYi. When I looked him up, I saw he was connected to Chen Xiaowang, the top family grandmaster of the family that created Tai Chi! That Ren came from mainland China was a big deal to me, because I was looking for this specific connection to China, especially since I grew up watching Kung Fu films.

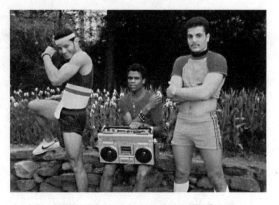

José (far left) as a break dancer in his pre–Tai Chi days

Ren first taught at the Wudang Martial Arts Academy in Flushing, Queens. He was new to the country and didn't know a lot about our customs. He put his early students under a lot of physical and mental stress to see who was worthy of sticking with the group. Ren had a way of weeding people out by testing their mettle. And that was a way for him to indoctrinate them into the "eating bitter" of traditional martial arts training. Most of us had martial arts backgrounds. But Ren was a force of nature. To see his strength, power, and beauty combined in one martial artist put us in awe.

I met Lou around '07 in Manhattan on the Hudson River. Ren and I were doing a trailer for a film idea I had. As the filming wrapped, Lou and Laurie visited the location. Lou had a real sense of joy watching Ren move and what we were doing.

When Ren started to perform with Lou, I told Ren, "If you ever did something more with Tai Chi, this would be a way to do it." Tai Chi is not presented as creatively as it could be. So when Stephan, Ren, and Lou came together to explore how to combine everything to present Tai Chi more creatively, the film *Final Weapon* came about.

I served as the line producer, so I pulled together a very experienced crew in Minnesota, where we shot the film. The talented cinematographer I recruited was skeptical. He said, "Wait a minute. You're saying Lou Reed is coming to Minnesota to do this film? Velvet Underground Lou Reed?" The next day Lou walks into my Tai Chi school in St. Paul, with Ren and Stephan. Everybody, especially the cinematographer, Sam Fisher, said, "Oh my God, I can't believe that's Lou Reed!" And then of course Lou was very cool and hugged everyone.

I showed the film crew a reel of Hong Kong martial arts films starring Donnie Yen, Stephan, and Hong Kong film legend Mike Woods. We had a real Hong Kong action team in Minnesota with a real-life rock and roll legend and an authentic martial arts master doing this really cool thing that we pulled off in just two days!

Day two of filming was when Lou took it all in. He smiled whenever he saw what Ren saw and was trying to do in the film. And I think the friendship they had, trying to help and support each other that weekend, really came through. Lou would walk around and observe everything quietly. He asked me quietly and politely, "José, do you mind if I take photos of the set?" In my head, I'm saying, *You're Lou Reed and this is your production too. Of course you can take pictures!* But I knew he was being genuine. Whenever he saw something interesting, he would smile and take a photo, like documenting secretly what he saw there.

During the production there were moments when we had a couple of times to quietly talk. One thing I remember was about their performance of "Sunday Morning" on the David Letterman show in 2004. In my ignorance, I asked Lou, "This is a beautiful song. Did you guys just record that?" And rather than correcting me, he said, "I recorded that years ago." He then smiled and placed his hand on my face like a father to his son and said, "José, the song is timeless."

WIM WENDERS

Film director

I must have met him before we did *Faraway, So Close!* That was in '92. He appeared in the film and gave a concert that we filmed, where he played one song for the shot.

We filmed in an industrial building out in what was then still the East. Berlin wasn't unified yet. The building was gigantic and had all this machinery still around. Really wild. Our character Cassiel was an angel

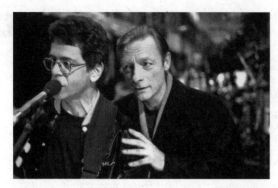
Lou Reed and Otto Sander in Faraway, So Close! *by Wim Wenders*

who had just become a human being, and one of the first things he does on his first day of life is he listens to Lou in his hotel. His first day in existence, and on his last day as an angel, he listens to Lou's thoughts. Later he sees a poster for a performance Lou is doing and goes and watches from the rafters. Lou selected "Why Can't I Be Good" to play for the scene. The tragedy of Cassiel, my angel, is that when he becomes a human being, he instantly gets into the wrong circles, and he sort of is involved with gangsters and goes down the drain very quickly, so "Why Can't I Be Good" was perfect.

He played the song three or four times. The shoot was finished, but the crowd was still there. Lou said, "Wait a minute, guys, I'll play you three more songs." And the crowd went wild. He did that because that crowd was so nice and they had all gone through the scene several times. We all gave up our shooting positions and just became the audience.

He was actually in three of my movies. He was also in *Palermo Shooting* and *The Soul of a Man*. In *Palermo Shooting* he plays a sort of ghost coming out of a jukebox, and in *Soul of a Man*, a film about my favorite blues musicians, he played a song by Skip James—"See That My Grave Is Kept Clean." An amazing song. And though I couldn't say that anybody is ever easy to work with, Lou made it always so easy. We never had a problem.

You know, I contributed a little story I wrote for a book called *The Songs of My Life*. My story was about "Pale Blue Eyes." It was a song that saved my life. It's a story about me in my revolutionary days in '68. I was living in a commune, traveled with all these people to Italy to meet these radical socialists. This was the moment when a lot of people I knew in Germany decided to go underground and start using violence. And some, like me, said, "No, we won't do that. We like our activities so far, and they are sort of fun and they are provocative, but nothing that would involve anybody getting hurt." Someone on the way home stole everything I had except my little tape recorder. I had one tape left and it was a Velvet Underground tape, and I listened to it over and over. That's where the story came from.

It was a terrible time for me. It was a time of great insecurity. Some of my best friends decided they were going to go and be part of something that I didn't want to be part of. Some died or disappeared, but I went back to being an art/film student and sort of disassociated myself from those revolutionary guys. "Some Kinda Love" and "Pale Blue Eyes" were running on a loop in my head. I didn't have anything else. It was his voice more than anything. He had this completely unique voice, like nobody else sang. This very charismatic, sort of rough and tender voice at the same time. It's what I liked most about the Velvets, Lou's voice. And when he was not singing, I thought they were not that great.

We met quite often, and Lou would always have to leave to do his Tai Chi. He spoke to me at length about this. He spoke of it very dearly. He thought I should do it, because I was complaining about getting stiff. He said, "Well, there's nothing better."

The only time I actually saw him do Tai Chi was when he stayed in Berlin. This was in early 2002, '03, '04? He said, "I can't practice in my hotel room. You know a place?" And I said, "Yes, I know the perfect place. We have a big gym in the house where I live. There's the gym and a swimming pool and a big flat area, and you're going to be totally on *He was* your own. Nobody is there ever during the day. You can have the whole *like an* place for yourself." I went along and did my own stuff at the gym, and Lou *angel* occupied this whole big area by the pool and was busy for about an hour. *dancing*

I was sweating on the treadmill and every now and again peeking *in this* over to what he was doing. I didn't want to sit there and watch him, but *big gym.* every now and then I looked, and he was very intensely working on it. It looked to me like he was defying gravity, and it looked to me like some ▲ of it was defying time, because everything was in slow motion. In a way, it was dance. It was beautiful. And he was like an angel dancing in this big gym and the sun was just falling through the windows.

ANOHNI

Singer, composer, visual artist, and vocalist with Lou's band on tour and on records

Hal Willner gave one of my CDs to Lou in 2001, while Lou was looking for some different kinds of guest vocalists for his album *The Raven*. It was one among a big pile of CDs, and Lou, for one reason or another, chose my voice out of all of those voices that he'd heard that day, and told Hal to

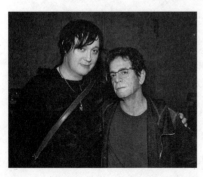
Anohni and Lou

bring me into the studio. Hal warned me that if Lou didn't like me that I would be escorted out of the studio through the back door, so he tried to prepare me, just in case anything bad happened. And I just went in. To be honest, I didn't know that much about Lou, and I'd been told that I was going to be trying to sing "Perfect Day." So I learned the song "Perfect

Day." I knew of Lou's work through people, through another generation of musicians who'd covered Lou's work, so it was strange in a way.

Anyway, I went in, and Lou liked what he heard, and he set up some candles for me. I was just along for the ride. I didn't have a lot of expectations. He liked me. It was thrilling to be liked by Lou. You immediately felt like you were someone special if Lou liked you. If Lou gave you his stamp, then you were in his psychic space and you were treasured.

He embraced my voice. I learned later about his history with the singer Jimmy Scott, and that also helped to shed light on what it was that Lou liked. He was taken by the meeting point between his incredibly rough voice and something more feminine . . . an androgynous voice that was supple. I think he was enchanted by that combination; he liked to have that energy around him, while he stayed his course.

And so in some ways, I think I filled a role that he'd explored, fleshed out, when he toured with Jimmy. But then I think we became friends because he saw in me a life experience that in some way he recognized. There was always this push and pull between the world that I came from, as someone who is transgender, and the broader society.

Lou's movement towards healthfulness is something that started long before I arrived . . . his movement towards a different kind of life, and a sort of shedding of, even a sort of silencing of, some parts of his story. At the same time, I felt he was drawn to me because I held space for certain points of view that were somehow magnetic for him.

He loved me, and I knew that, and I loved him. He understood something about the predicament I was in. This was the early 2000s, and the environment in music was particularly homophobic, particularly transphobic. So much has changed in the last fifteen years, it's hard to remember that there was literally no space for someone like me in music, and in popular culture. He once wrote a letter on the eve of the release of *The Raven* to Seymour Stein and it just said, "If there's one thing left for you to do in this life, it's sign Antony and the Johnsons."

Stein didn't sign me, but the fact was that he wrote that letter. . . . It was shocking to have someone like him, this kind of hyper-masculine tough guy whose bark was so loud, advocating for me.

Lou had a straight line to his power. There was a dam built between his power and his rage. And sometimes, depending on where he was psychically, that dam was in better or worse shape. Sometimes the dam would break. When he was in his grace, it was about building this new kind of composure and grace, reaching for this kind of deeper strengthening that worked for him. Especially in the last part of his life, when I knew him, it often really served him, not just in his practice but in his life in terms of being able to express the generosity and grace that was the essence of him. We all know Lou. We know the size of him. He had a lot on his plate.

Did his decision at that point in his life to defend a trans artist reflect on his previous relationships with transgender people? I think he would hate me for saying that. He would probably say, actually, "That's bullshit, I just liked you."

The Raven tour was a cavalcade. Lou had banned the drums; he hated drums at that point because he couldn't control them in the way he wanted. He had Mike Rathke on guitar, who also was asked to play this tiny electronic drum kit. It was very idiosyncratic.

But if we're talking about a straight line, the straight line was his emotional commitment. Everything fell to the wayside when Lou started to sing or started to deliver. Lou playing guitar—that was always my thing. I was always begging him, "Lou, please play the guitar," because often he didn't want to play. He would say, "I can't remember how to play anymore." And I'd say, "Lou, when you play the guitar, it's like a lion's paw clawing at a guitar. No one else sounds like that." It's just this intuitive way of playing that is so emotional. He was such a good guitar player.

And then of course when Master Ren came out and did Tai Chi, it was Lou daring the audience to challenge his values. "Just go ahead and don't embrace my values. See what happens next."

I remember sitting with him in a coffee shop on Perry Street and he was just so peaceful. He'd really arrived at this plateau of peace. And that was why his last album was such a shock. He channeled rage for his last record. I always see it in the context of the medical treatments he was dealing with at the time. Because it kind of boiled his blood from the in-side, when he was taking that interferon. It can be a very difficult treatment to endure, and it just changed him.

Lou had a straight line to his power.

▲

But I remember so well the stability of his spirit, prior to those treat-ments. He was in a place of graciousness that evolved during the years that I knew him. When I was first on tour with him, he was still full of grit. If his steak was too tough, or if something was going wrong on tour, a head had to roll. Someone would say the wrong thing to Master Ren, and Lou would fire the cook. So many cooks' heads rolled on that tour. He could be volatile and mercurial. You didn't always know what to expect.

Ren was a different kind of tough. I think Lou loved Ren because Ren's story was so hard-knock. He was sleeping on a concrete bench as a young apprentice. Ren had mastered his demons through training, sheer force of will, and mental control. I think that idea of mental control really appealed to Lou.

It wasn't "Dive into the ocean and let it carry you." It was like "Build a fortress and lock it down." And within that, "Find your own line that connects you down into the center of the earth." And that was what Ren exhibited every night onstage. He would do these dances. . . . Lou was obsessed with the idea that Ren could basically knock over a building if his mind was set on it, almost like a bulldozer or a battering ram. I think Lou was drawn to this idea that if a mind was clear enough and perfectly aligned with its body, it could move a mountain. That power impressed him, but I think it also appealed to his desire to be the master of his life, and of the things that had happened to him, and to the oceans of feeling, power, confusion, and expression that poured through him.

He felt life really intensely. He was a deeply feeling person. He cried from the tiny peep of a violin. He was so emotional, and so receptive, and that stood in dramatic contrast to his volatility. So he's dealing with this huge spectrum of tenderness and intensity, and it was Tai Chi that drew all of those strands together, into a person that felt self-actualized, self-realized. It gave him authorship over the spectrum of his experience.

He'd put in the time, he'd invested the time, he'd done the work, and he had it in the bank, and that was what gave him access to such grace. That foundation of grace that he'd achieved did carry him through, especially through the last months of his life, when he was really shining.

But I remembered the same tenderness from before the interferon treatments, a few years earlier . . . because he'd already gotten there on his own. Before he was dealing with his mortality so explicitly, he'd gotten there. He had gotten to his grace. And then he got assaulted with medical stuff.

When we talk about the metaphor of the straight line, I think there were certain straight lines in his crazy life, within all his complexity. . . . This sheer force of will, I think, was ultimately what he embraced as his straight line, and what drew him to this notion of mastery, more than to surrender. It was really mastery that offered a kind of a solution to him.

I remember even the last time I had dinner with him, he was telling me, "You've got to get it together." I miss him so much, because life is lonely

Most people aren't very alive. They don't feel that much. Lou would make you feel.

▲

without those people that feel so deeply the experience of living. Lou was one of those people that when you're with him, you're with someone who is really alive. Most people aren't very alive. They don't feel that much. Lou would make you feel. No matter whether you felt claustrophobic or you were laughing or you were a little frightened, or fascinated, or whatever feeling you were having next to Lou, you knew that you were alive next to Lou.

I made a post when he died that said he was like a father to me. My own father probably would've acknowledged that. Lou died shortly before my dad died, but Lou had mentored me. He saw what was beautiful in me and wanted it, in stark contrast to how my own father dealt with me.

So Lou knew what I was, and he tried to protect me. Sometimes when parents are protecting children, they crush parts of them that they're worried will make life more difficult. It's classic and paradoxical. He knew where I wanted to go and used all of his faculties and resources to try to make that happen. That my life transformed so dramatically and that I developed a platform—these were both in large part because of Lou.

I think of Hal's pile of CDs. Had he just skipped over that CD, none of this would've happened. That's so bizarre.

LAURIE ANDERSON: It would've happened. It would've happened in another way. There's no way that people can't hear your music.

ANOHNI: But I was thirty-five when that happened. I'd been banging on doors for well over a decade. Everyone had said no. Lou turned the no around. It wasn't just, "We haven't heard you yet." It was like, "We've heard you and we are saying no. We're not going to let this pass through the doors into the daylight of popular culture." Lou was the one who pried that door open for me. He reorganized all these straight guys to listen to me through Lou's ears. Lou gave tough guys permission to cry when they heard me sing.

He was an artist. He embodied creativity and suffering, and a very, very fierce life force.

He'd just been through a lot more hell than most people. So when you've been through a lot more hell than most people, you just have different skill sets. Most people couldn't fathom his life experience. Sometimes we make artists of those individuals; we marvel over them. They're like these weird pearls that our culture has made. You know, our society mulches people's spirits, and then the ones that survive turn into these glistening pearls, and then we're fascinated by them, because they contain this depth of experience, especially if they start to express themselves in these transcendental ways. It shocks people. It shocks the heterosexual experience. It disrupts the performance of suffering complacency that most people are forced to exhibit in daily life. Lou just had a very vivid life. He experienced vivid joy and vivid suffering, and from very early on he was burned into the form that was him. Sometimes he was a mountain of scar tissue. And flowering, he was flowering.

LAURIE: Yeah, he was a flower.

ANOHNI: What does it take for scar tissue to flower? Nina Simone has it in her song "Compassion," where she talks about . . . creativity. It's a real gift, especially for those who have suffered. She says, "Because I have loved so deeply . . . God, in his great compassion, gave me the gift of song." It's about survival.

Creativity is available to us all, but it is a rare thing when a child feels that they have permission—for one reason or another—to reach for their creativity as a means of survival, whatever it is that they're enduring. When that neural pathway opens in our society, which mostly tells children to shut up, when a child for one reason or another reaches for self-expression, if only in secrecy, to compensate in some way for what they've endured, then you get a lighthouse.

The second part of the lyric is "Because I have loved so vainly, sung with such faltering breath." Nina talks about her depth of feeling as a reason that God gave her song. Finally, she talks about her depth of singing as the reason "the master in his infinite mercy, offers the boon of death." It's just a very amazing lyric. It's talking about being like a soldier of God, or a soldier of creativity. I see God and creativity as interchangeable.

I think 2006 was a golden period for Lou, going into the restaging of *Berlin*. Doing *Berlin* was such a point of joy for him. I'll never forget how happy he was. He really reached the mountaintop when that *New York Times* article came out, and Lou was celebrated for a crucial piece of his work that had previously been defiled in the media. Lou was the one that helped me to understand that a malevolent media assault on an artist can create PTSD. When you get assaulted that publicly, really, it's a kind of violence. An artist can be thrown into the coliseum and recreationally shat upon in front of millions of people. It's a sacrifice to appease the collective hunger for a misplaced moment of revenge. It is part of who we have become as a species, and another indication of our collective brokenness as a society.

LAURIE: We were talking to Bill Berger who was his tour manager and lighting designer a little while ago. He was just talking about Lou crying. He said, in the airport he had read a couple of really bad reviews of his work, and that he was crying. And that really shocked me, because he seemed, in many ways, so secure.

ANOHNI: Oh God, wasn't he the opposite? Even one negative word would upset him. If it was only four stars, it was an assault. Lou carried trauma from previous assaults, and that's why he couldn't actually endure one word. I can relate to that. When you have been publicly shamed by people who wish the worst for you, in exchange for a little bit of money from your actual fans, and that's the final extent of the transaction . . . as if a little pile of money from those who appreciate your work gives the rest of the world license to say whatever they want about you, no matter how biased or personally defamatory. That happened to Lou, and reached an apex with the initial release of *Berlin*.

When he was talking about restaging *Berlin*, Lou initially wanted me to sing that whole show, and that wasn't a fleeting idea. He wanted *Berlin* to happen, but he did not want to sing the show. It took many dinners for me to convince him. I said, "Lou, no one wants to hear me sing *Berlin*. People will just be frustrated. Everyone wants to hear you sing *Berlin*." He's like, "No, no, I can't sing those songs." I don't know, but I think he was traumatized by the earlier rejection of that work, and his gut reaction was not to risk it again.

So then he got up the courage, the band pulled together, the orchestra, it got more and more exciting. He was living inside the cocoon of the work being restaged, and it sounded so good, because that album is *so good*. It's one of the great albums of the twentieth century. But he was so fucked over with the reviews of that album that he did *Metal Machine Music* next, which is basically just like: "I hate you. All I can feel is my hatred for you. All I can feel is my rejection of all your judgment of me. I annihilate your rejection." You know what I mean? I'm not saying *Metal Machine Music* didn't have musical merit; of course it did have tremendous musical merit. But I feel like I understand the impulse to try to annihilate a culture's rejection of you as an artist. Your only remaining agency is to try to build a wall high enough to prevent that toxicity from soaking into your psyche.

Yoko Ono once told me that when John Lennon was shot, the second bullet that hit the window was meant for her. And in the aftermath, the whole society, internationally, blamed her for the end of the Beatles, and even for his death; people expressed so much hatred for her at that point of such terrible loss in her own life. And she said, "My solution to it was to imagine that the energy that was hitting me was a form of universal love." What kind of strength of will does that take, to reimagine a diseased and overwhelming assault upon you as an impersonal flow of love from the universe? It was such a brilliant and visionary concept, in response to the tragic ways that we treat each other.

Lou had his own way of dealing with it. This is a long way of saying that when we staged *Berlin*, it was so beautiful, and that glowing *New York Times* article came out, and it was a game changer. This time Lou was celebrated for being a pioneer. His contribution to culture was reassessed, thirty years later. The paper of note acknowledged that he had given something of himself to the world and taken a risk on everyone's behalf.

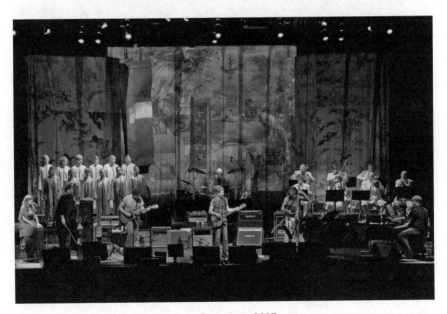

Berlin *tour, 2007*

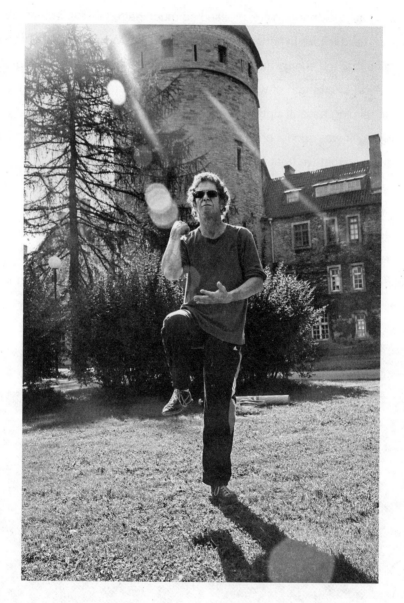

Practicing on tour in Europe, mid-2000s

CHAPTER 8

TAI CHI ON TOUR

Hey man, what's your style?

BILL BERGER

Tour manager and lighting designer, late '90s–2000s

Once hotel security was put on alert because someone reported this weird guy in the courtyard swinging a sword. It was Lou doing Tai Chi. Really, if you look out from your hotel window and you see a guy just swinging a sword, it's a concern. Also, having metal swords in a wardrobe case just isn't a really great thing to try and deal with on tour.

Lou always required a room large enough for him to practice Tai Chi or access to a small ballroom or gym for that purpose. It was a very, very, very important thing. And he also didn't like to see cranes outside his window. "I don't want to see construction." Foremost, though, was he needed a space for Tai Chi.

Master Ren and I got along great. "Master Ren, here's where you stand onstage, because I have a special light. Master Ren?" He's smiling at me. Does he know what I'm saying? "I have focused a special light for you downstage right. So when you come out, I will have a mark on it, a little X. You stand there, and you'll be in perfect light." Whenever Master Ren came onstage, I would reduce the rest of the lighting and would give Master Ren, as Lou wanted it, the attention during those songs. Master Ren knew what I said. He knew where the light was. I don't think he ever missed his mark, regardless of where we were, or if it was a super-wide stage, or a smaller stage, wherever that spike mark was. It's not like you could see him looking for it. He would be facing Lou, and then he'd face the audience, the music would start, and he would start.

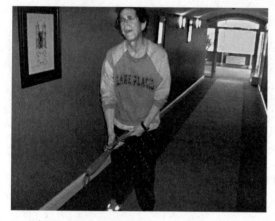

Lou took his weapons on tour

Master Ren was always smiling, but no smiles when he was performing. It was pretty amazing. My place was front of house. He'd start, and many times I'd see audience heads turning toward each other, like, *What the hell is this?* You come for Lou Reed and rock and roll, and this guy comes out in pajamas and starts doing stuff onstage. It never failed. But by the time he came out the second time, it worked. You didn't see the heads turning. Well, maybe a couple, like, *Not again*.

We were doing a show in Modena with a lot of other artists, and Lou asked, "Could I meet James Brown?" who was also performing. I went to his manager, and when I mentioned Lou's request, James just lit up. I have a picture of them like two kids.

And for the other side of that experience, we were playing Neil Young's Bridge School Benefit, and Metallica was playing as well. Kirk Hammett, their guitarist, approached me out in the courtyard where all these portable dressing rooms were around and asked, "Do you think I could meet Mr. Reed?" Lou was delighted. And to Kirk Hammett it was, "Oh, no, no, call me Lou." This was the first time he dealt with Metallica. Later on, they played together at the twenty-fifth anniversary of the Rock and Roll Hall of Fame. Out of that came the idea of Metallica doing a "best of" Lou Reed album. Which I thought was sensational. They didn't make that but finally did the album *Lulu* together.

Lou was invited to the White House when Václav Havel, former Czech president, was a guest. They were having a state dinner, and the policy was whomever the guest asked for would be invited. Havel said, "I want Lou Reed." Okay, this was, like, two weeks after Monica Lewinsky.

Someone at the White House wanted a set list. I submitted a list that included "Dirty Blvd." Lou always wanted to include "Sex with Your Parents" in the list, but that's another story. Well, the White House calls. "Mr. Berger, I received the set list you emailed me, and we're having some issues." I said, "What would that be?" She said, "Well, 'Dirty Blvd.,' in particular." "Well, what is the issue there?" "Tipper Gore's going to be there, and it's a state dinner. And of course you know about recent events at the White House

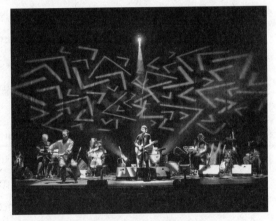

Onstage with Ren, 2003

in the past couple of weeks—well, that song won't be appropriate." I said, "What in particular in that song?" She said, "I don't know the exact line. It's something about the whores calling the cops out for a suck. There might be more to it than that, but the whores calling the cops out for a suck." I said, "When you said that, it really didn't sound that bad." "Well, okay. . . ."

He did the song and I remember being in the room, there is Tipper hitting her thighs to the beat of "Dirty Blvd.," and there's Kissinger sitting with Mia Farrow, and the president and the First Lady and the vice president just enjoying the song, and Lou sings, "The TV whores are calling the cops out for a suck," and it was all fine.

CHUCK HAMMER

Musician, composer, founder of Guitarchitecture, and guitarist for Lou Reed from the late '70s to the early '80s

As it turns out, I studied Tai Chi briefly in '76—prior to working with Lou in '78—and in fact may have actually and inadvertently been his initial early contact with it. I met Lou initially in November '78. I flew in from Santa Barbara for an audition, after writing Lou a letter, which to my surprise he actually answered with a direct phone call. I was studying Tai Chi out there in '77. I only remember mentioning it to Lou during our first New York City rehearsals February to March '79.

It seemed somewhat inconsequential at the time. He mentioned that he had hurt his back and was trying to get in shape for the tour. That was the actual context at the time. What happened prior to March '79 regarding Lou and Tai Chi, I do not know. However, in March '79 he purchased a wooden roller pin for his back. I first saw it riding up to rehearsal in an elevator with him near St. Mark's Place. It was his rehearsal space at the time, called Star Sound on Lafayette Street. When I saw the roller, I mentioned that I had used one similar while studying Tai Chi.

At the time, Lou never mentioned it again, but I was surprised when he displayed an interest in martial arts films. We watched that film *The 36th Chamber of Shaolin* in a theater in Lisbon. This outwardly had nothing per se to do with Tai Chi, but there was a definite philosophical edge to that film that resonated in a related direction.

TONY "THUNDER" SMITH

Drummer, singer, composer, and professor at Berklee College of Music; drummer for Lou from 1995 to 2013

I had worked with so many different musicians and leaders, and Lou knew what he wanted, and it was great to work with him. I started working with him on the *Set the Twilight Reeling* record. After that record was done, we went out as a trio. It was Lou, myself, Fernando, and we did some shows in London, and then a little while later Mike Rathke came on board and then it was just a quartet. We were a team doing gigs, doing whatever Lou wanted to do, whether it was in New York or whether it was in Europe. It was just fast moving—we did a lot of shows.

Before we went onstage, we would put our hands in. When the last person got their hand on top, then we would move it up and down and up and down, until it was kind of like pumping yourselves up, and

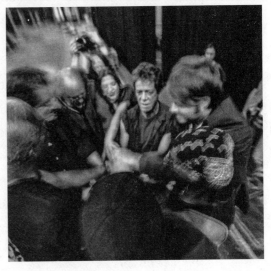

we used to do that after or before every gig. It just happened, and it carried on, and when Mama Ruth passed, we added Mama Ruth's name in the mix.

Mama Ruth would go on tour with us because it would be very strenuous for Lou—Mama Ruth would just take care of Lou and make sure that with the acupuncture and the deep-tissue massage and everything, he was ready to

Band gets up for the show

go, and it could spill over into everybody in the group. It was like, okay, well, Lou would go, "Okay, Tony. Ruth, go to Tony, go to Fernando." It became a thing where she always kept us so healthy. The first time Mama Ruth gave me acupuncture, I didn't see the big deal until I tried to get up off the floor afterwards. I couldn't move—I was stuck to the floor. I mean, then I got up, I was amazed. I said, "Wow! Unbelievable—the stuff really works!" Mama Ruth was absolutely amazing, and she was such a character. She used to carry a rice-cooking pot on the road and cook up healthy things for us.

I could see for Lou that doing Tai Chi was a very personal thing. I had been, then, involved in Nichiren Shōshū Buddhism and I understood—I kind of understood—everything is just as personal as somebody saying, "Hey, you need to go down to the Buddhist temple." You know what I mean? "Let me take you to the Buddhist temple." If it's something that works for you, and it's very private, then you leave it that way unless somebody else that you know expresses an interest.

I loved Master Ren—he's just amazing. You'd really never think that Master Ren does what he does. He's such a character. I remember one time we went out to a Chinese restaurant—we were on tour and it was just like he was the king. He was ordering everything for everybody, he wouldn't let anybody speak. It was beautiful food, and he had kind of sussed everybody out and he knew what everybody eats. Watching Master Ren onstage, I saw the power, and it was thrilling for me as a drummer because it was very, very percussive. When he landed on the stage, it would sound like a huge bass drum and thunder. It was thrilling, and to watch him do his forms, you know—I mean, wow!

When Master Ren would come on tour, he and Lou would practice and do forms outside, they would do forms on the roof and/or in his hotel room, but they were always doing Tai Chi. There was not a day where he wasn't doing Tai Chi. I said, "Wow, man, Lou is in such great shape, and he's always doing this and he's always full of energy."

BETH GROUBERT

Personal assistant to Lou, mid-'90s

Lou had this great camaraderie with all the guys that were touring with him. He really seemed to love it. If the tour people, the promoters, wanted to take him out to dinner, Lou would always say, "Only if the entire crew can come." He always made sure everybody was taken care of, and he would also stay to himself at times. Sometimes Lou would disappear during the daytime and do his own thing. In 1996, on tour in Japan, I do remember setting up time for him to practice Tai Chi in his hotel.

Once in Japan he wasn't feeling well and something was going on. He was feeling a little speedy. He goes, "Don't get it. I don't understand this. I've just been drinking green tea all day long and I'm feeling really wired." I said, "Lou, green tea has tons of caffeine." And he says, "It does?" And I said, "Yes." Very funny. He said, "For crying out loud, I always find speed wherever I go."

KEVIN HEARN

Member of Barenaked Ladies, musical director for Lou in the 2000s

Well, I first met Lou over the phone. I think in 2000. I was visiting the Reprise Records head office in Los Angeles, and Howie Klein always sort of gave us the latest CDs that were just about to come out. So I asked Howie Klein if he had the latest Lou Reed CD, which was . . . I think *Ecstasy* was just about to come out. And he said, "Oh, are you a Lou fan?" I said,

"Oh yeah, he's been my hero most of my life." So he said, "Lou's a good friend of mine," and took out the phone and dialed Lou's number and introduced us. I told Lou how much his work had meant to me all through my life. Then I said, "I hope you don't mind me saying that." And he said, "Oh no, it's always nice and reassuring when someone says something like that." And he said, "Congratulations on all your success." That was about it. I figured I'd never hear from him again, or talk to him again.

Months later, I became ill; I was diagnosed with cancer and had to have a bone marrow transplant. I was in really bad shape. Too weak to even lift up a telephone or go up and down stairs. I received an email from Lou, out of the blue, that said, "Hey, Kevin, it's Lou. I hear you're not doing well. I hope you get better real soon and get back to your music."

There he is.

It meant the world to me at the time. That was the first day I was strong enough to walk around the block. Just 'cause I felt so inspired by Lou's kindness. He didn't need to do that. He didn't really know me. Yeah, it's a very special memory.

A bit later, Lou invited me down for a show at the Knitting Factory. I was just well enough to make the trip from Toronto at that point. I was still thin, and I still have the photo of me and Lou. I remember he held my hand and said, "Kevin, you must have balls of steel." Which I thought was such a funny thing—here he was just eating pistachios, and it was my first entrance into Lou's world, where you look around the room and there's Philip Glass and Neil Young and you [Laurie], Fernando. Just meeting all those people was a real thrill. Then Lou invited me for pizza, which I couldn't believe.

I think this would have been the late '90s, and I remember I was saying goodbye to Mike Rathke and Jeremy Darby and walking towards the entrance, and I heard Lou's voice say, "We're waiting for Kevin." We got in the car, and it was me, and Lou, you [Laurie], in the back seat. That's the first time that we met and went out.

I made a record after my cancer treatment, kind of about the whole thing, and I sent a copy to Lou, who wrote back and said, "Kevin, you've made something beautiful. You've gone somewhere most people don't come back from and you've reported on it."

When I first started playing with the band, Stewart Hurwood and Mike Rathke both warned me, if Lou shouts, it's nothing personal, just don't shout back, and I remember, every single thing I did, Lou was watching me like crazy. I remember I was going to step on the distortion pedal, 'cause I was going to do a lead, and right before my foot hit the pedal, he said, "Don't." Or rehearsing "Satellite of Love," I thought, *I'm gonna make some white noise, open the filter, and do a little* [*makes white noise sound*], so he stops the band. "What was that, Kevin? A rocket ship?" He said, "Don't do that."

Another one was "Sweet Jane." I started playing the organ melody that happens in the outro, and he stopped the band. He goes, "Were you playing that organ melody?" I said, "Yes, I was, Lou." He goes, "No one's played that in a million years." I said, "That's a long time." And he said, "Yes, and for good reason."

There's the other side too. I thought, *I'm going to play celeste on "Pale Blue Eyes," just a nice bell sound*. And he stopped the band and he goes, "Kevin, you're a fucking mind reader. I love that." So it wasn't always, you know . . . It was both. When we took a break, he said, "Kevin, I hope you don't mind the way I work; some people don't like it." And I said, "Lou, I'm here for you, I'm here to try to help you with your vision. How can I do that if you don't tell me what you like, or don't like?" He made me the band leader soon after that.

SCOTT RICHMAN: I remember you were bringing new songs to the repertoire that maybe he hadn't thought about performing for a long time.

KEVIN HEARN: I tried to keep all of Lou's music in mind to play on tour. I remember I'd play a song—it was "I Remember You," I think—and he said, "How do you know that? No one knows that song except you, me, and seven seagulls." He was so funny.

We played a show for the Whitney in a tent somewhere. We're just doing a trio with Lou. It's me, Sarth, Rob Wasserman, and Lou. We were going to do "Walk on the Wild Side." And we're running through it at rehearsal, and he's working with Rob on the bass line and asks me to just play acoustic guitar. So I'm just cycling through those two chords, over and over again—it must have been about twenty-five minutes—while he worked on the bass line with Rob. I just sort of started drifting off and playing it. Then he turned to me and said, "There, that, you finally played it right." I'm like, "Oh." Yeah. Like . . . he was . . . You know what I mean, right? And he was always telling me to relax, even onstage. He'd come over and whisper and say, "Kevin, relax."

He seemed particularly keen on talking to me every show. He would come over and say something to me. I'd be playing piano and he'd come over and say, "That's too smart." Or he'd come over, and I was really into playing, and he'd come over and say, "Stand up straight." One night he came over and said, "I couldn't do this without you."

We had our little moments every night onstage, and I play in a band where we talk a lot onstage and joke around with each other. It's kind of a sparring match sometimes, in a comedic way. One night we were doing the song "I'm Sticking with You." And I added a flourish at the end on the piano, and Lou said, "Oh, Kevin, I liked that. I wish that was on the record." I'm just so used to talking onstage with my bandmates, and I said, "Well, Lou, I would have played it on your record, but I wasn't born yet."

The rest of the band looked at me like, *What are you doing? You idiot.* And every night after that, when he introduced that song, it became this thing. He'd go, "Some of you might remember this song, some of you might not have been born yet." He'd look back at me. So we had this sort of comfort together onstage that I think he appreciated.

He didn't want to do the old things. He kept renewing them, creating new ways of doing his music that was really, really adventurous. So many people just stick to their formulas, and he didn't do that.

And it is amazing he gave me a chance. I remember he used to say, "Kevin, when Laurie does a show, she doesn't do old songs. Every time it's new." I think he was trying to find a middle ground somehow. When we did do old material, he'd always want to reinvent it. It had to feel fresh.

In 2013, we were going to do Coachella, but instead we ended up at the Cleveland Clinic.

It was full circle in a way—he wrote to me when I was really sick. He called me and said, "Kevin, I've been diagnosed with something I know you're familiar with, and would you mind if I called you sometimes just to vent or, you know, see what you think?" And I said, "That'd be an absolute honor." And he said, "I might just be calling you to tell you they chopped one of my nuts off and chucked it in the Hudson River."

And then he called and told me about the new speaker system he bought. "'Cause when I croak, I'm gonna have good sound." Even then our friendship became richer and deeper, and quite bittersweet because, yeah, he was dying. It was an honor to be at the Cleveland Clinic. I went whenever I could, I did. I stayed in the room next door.

LAURIE ANDERSON: He was really making such an effort. Part of this book is about how Tai Chi, meditation, and just general nerve help you face sickness and your own death.

KEVIN: I remember they had a deck on the roof of the clinic; Lou loved going up there. I took him there for a bit of sun and air and a look at the sky, and he would close his eyes and meditate. I helped him to lie down on the deck. After a moment, he said, "What are you doing, standing up there?" I lay down next to him. That was what it was like—that's what it was like with Lou.

STEWART HURWOOD

Lou's guitar technician 2003–2013

I started working for Lou in 2003, '04. I got a call from Bill Berger, saying, "I've heard your name. Are you interested in touring with Lou Reed?" Most of the crew had just been fired or quit. Because of that situation, nothing was festival ready. I said yes. We started getting it together, and eventually the band came in. Then Lou came in. I didn't know much about him, I wasn't a fan of his, but when he showed up, he had a lot of presence and energy. He walked over to me and said, "I hear you're a fan of color coding. Me too. Welcome aboard."

I was the tech for Lou, Mike, and Fernando then, and they had me running ragged. I was working eighteen-hour days, getting it all together. For me, it's "What's wrong? Let's fix it." You shouldn't ever try to figure out what Lou's thinking, but I had to. But Lou did love it when I tried to think ahead and anticipate problems and his needs. That's how it all started.

Touring with him was different. We were in Australia, I believe, and somebody from the promoter asked if there was anything he'd like. He responded, "Yes, I want Chinese weaponry from the sixteenth century." They would go off shopping.

Tai Chi and Master Ren were there from the beginning. Lou was very much into Tai Chi and its promotion. We would be doing a show, and Ren would come out onstage in these flowing red robes and perform with the band. My job was to watch Lou. He was watching Ren.

Master Ren on tour was my introduction to Tai Chi, but I saw more when touring with Metal Machine Trio [MM3]. It's a very complex show, with the drone guitars, Lou, Ulrich Krieger, and Sarth Calhoun playing and all being mixed with the drones and live samples. The first performance was at REDCAT in LA. They put everything into the show, and after, we're completely spent, emotionally gone, and had to do a second show in twenty minutes. Lou said, "Sarth, let's do Push Hands." He said to me, "When you do this, you're pulling in energy from the universe. It's coming through you and it's energizing you." I couldn't argue with him because I just witnessed it. I just saw it with my own eyes. That happened. It was real. They had no energy, then they had plenty. They didn't drink or eat, they just did Push Hands.

Once I was moving equipment after a show and Lou came in the next day and said, "You need to do Tai Chi. You're a natural. Yesterday you did a move that was perfect. You just did it. People train to do that, and you just did it."

Since the MM3 tour, Lou has always ended shows with the drones. "I feel held in the drones," he would say. The most fun moments with Lou were when we were experimenting with the drones. He was as excited as a five-year-old.

A show I remember well was in Brighton. It was in the Spire, which is an old, disused church. Beautiful stained-glass windows. We had the lights going, and six guitars. I always use different tunings. I have different compositions and ideas to start, but at some point, I'm going to fly. If something feels good, you hold with that for a while before moving on. At the New York Public Library show it was cool to play really loud where loud usually isn't. I would love to play more.

The success of *Berlin* in 2006 was a huge change for him. He finally got the attention and the confirmation of his genius after taking thirty years of terrible shit for the same thing. Then he had the same belated response to *Metal Machine Music*. Lou had done so much and was now getting the respect. He got younger guys in the band. He had a new attitude—more open and less intimidating. It was great to see.

I still feel pissed off that he's dead.

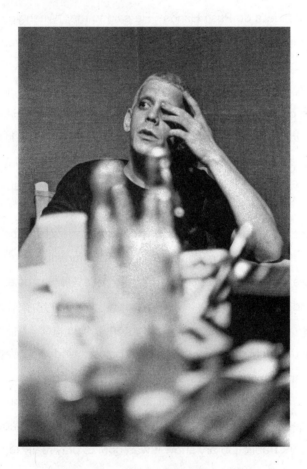

Photo of Lou on tour, by Mick Rock, 1974

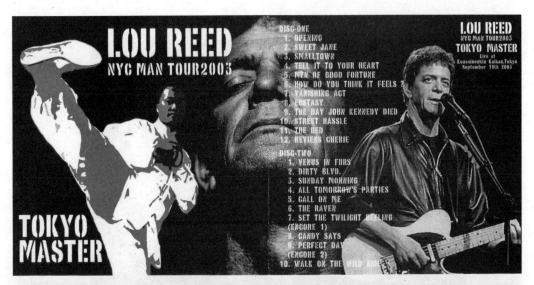

LOU REED
NYC MAN TOUR 2003

TOKYO MASTER

DISC-ONE
1. OPENING
2. SWEET JANE
3. SMALLTOWN
4. TELL IT TO YOUR HEART
5. MEN OF GOOD FORTUNE
6. HOW DO YOU THINK IT FEELS ?
7. VANISHING ACT
8. ECSTASY
9. THE DAY JOHN KENNEDY DIED
10. STREET HASSLE
11. THE BED
12. REVIEN CHERIE
DISC-TWO
1. VENUS IN FURS
2. DIRTY BLVD.
3. SUNDAY MORNING
4. ALL TOMORROW'S PARTIES
5. CALL ON ME
6. THE RAVEN
7. SET THE TWILIGHT REELING
(ENCORE 1)
8. CANDY SAYS
9. PERFECT DAY
(ENCORE 2)
10. WALK ON THE WILD SIDE

LOU REED
NYC MAN TOUR 2003
TOKYO MASTER
Live at
Kouseinenkin Kaikan,Tokyo
September 19th 2003

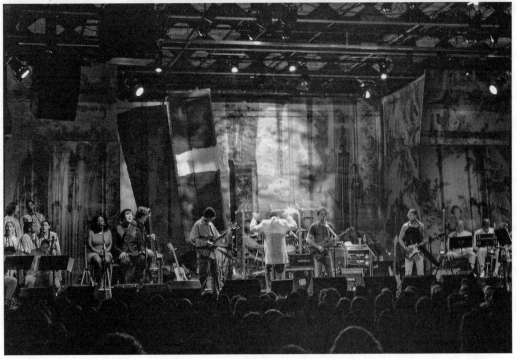

Above: Bootleg CD from Japanese tour, 2003; below: Berlin *stage*

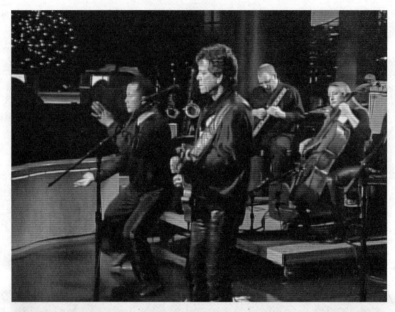

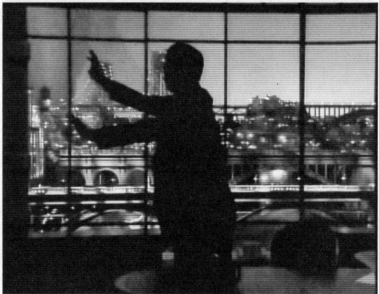

"What do you do in the dark when your guests are singing onstage," asks a viewer of
The Late Show's *David Letterman? Naturally, Letterman practices alongside Lou and Master
Ren who performed "Sunday Morning" in February 2004 on his CBS program.*

CHAPTER 9

TAI CHI IN PUBLIC

Just say "go" and that is that, I'm a New York City man

From an unedited interview with Lou by Tracee Hutchison for The 7.30
Report, *2007, included in* Rage: Tribute to Lou Reed, *TV special, ABC1
(Australia TV), November 2, 2013*

TRACEE HUTCHISON: It's been really important to you, the Tai Chi—
what brought you and what led you to it?

LOU REED: It's too complicated to go into, but I always wanted to do
an exercise that was good for something besides being exercise. I mean
if being an auto mechanic was actually healthy for you, maybe I'd have
done that.

TRACEE: It's a combination of the physical and the mental.

LOU: And the spiritual. It's everything. . . .

TRACEE: I do Yoga so I guess that's how I get out of my busy head sometimes, so I wonder whether or not that was an attraction for you.

LOU: It's that it's beautiful.

TRACEE: A beautiful thing to perform.

LOU: A beautiful thing to do in every conceivable way, and will teach you
about your body, will improve your body. It can transform your body into
something you didn't know perhaps that you had. The fact that it goes
back hundreds and hundreds and hundreds of years—these people were
very smart and they put together this system that was good for health and
also to protect yourself, and you can do it till you're 112. It's not just the
old people in the park.

There's power in this. They call it "fajin." I'm just saying most people,
they think of Tai Chi, they think of very old people doing it very slow. Not

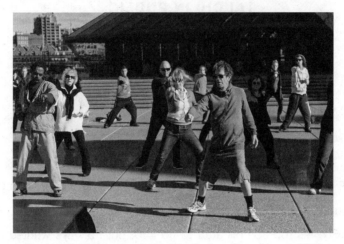

Teaching Tai Chi on the steps of the Sydney Opera House, 2010

Chen Tai Chi, which is the first system. When other people left this system, they were able to leave it, but they had to leave certain parts out. It's the parts they left out that I like. Typically. . . . And I'll tell you one other thing: some doctor friends of mine have told me people they see most with knee problems are Yoga people.

TRACEE: My knees are fine. . . .

LOU: Beautiful and in shape.

TRACEE: I'm doing okay. I know it's tiresome for you to revisit the tales of rock 'n' roll excesses, the walks on the wild side, and now the big rock 'n' roll story is really about sobriety.

LOU: Well, don't even bother with that side.

TRACEE: I'm wondering what sobriety has shown you, though.

LOU: What did I just say to you? This was not one of those questions that was submitted, so forget it.

TRACEE: Can I ask you, then, do you see a time when you don't want to be doing this anymore?

LOU: One of the things we wanted to do in New York City was open a Tai Chi school where you also had meditation, and we're friends with some people who are fairly well known in what they do—like Mingyur Rinpoche—who wrote a book called *The Joy of Living*. I study with him and certain herbalists, and we thought it would be really great to have this all centered in one place. That's something I'd love to have something to do with. I'd love to go to China as a photographer of martial arts. I mean I'm really good at that because I know what to look for.

GENE CHING

Publisher of Kung Fu Tai Chi *magazine, staff writer for YMAA Publication Center, and Shaolin Temple martial arts disciple*

I'm a lifelong practitioner of Chinese martial arts. Not so much Tai Chi, though I have done a bit. Unlike Lou, I'm not a Chen-style practitioner, though I have great respect for the form. In fact my name in Chinese is actually the character for Chen.

All forms of Tai Chi are Chuan, or "fist," arts, meaning martial arts. And Chen Tai Chi preserves that in many ways, more overtly than any of the other Tai Chi styles. It's really clear.

Chen is a big topic. There are many people talking and writing about it. Master Ren was a major force in this, actually. Chen is very rigorous, and it's not what most people expect Tai Chi to be, especially in the West. The explosiveness is just hard for people to wrap their heads around. I think most Americans, when they think of Tai Chi, are actually thinking of Chi gong.

I met Lou as publisher of *Kung Fu Tai Chi* magazine. He was a student of Master Ren's, whom we had worked with previously. Master Ren brought Lou to meet us.

My first meeting with Lou was a bit rough. I hadn't prepared. But once I began talking about a beautiful animated photo sequence of Tai Chi that a number of Ren's students had made, it became easier. After that, we had a pretty good conversation about Tai Chi and music, among other things. Lou knew his stuff. He was well read. I think the problem that a lot of people in the martial arts have is they just take what their master says without question. But Lou wasn't like that at all. He studied and practiced.

You could make a very strong argument that Tai Chi is the most popular martial art in the world. It has a huge following, including many seniors. If you go to China, you will see hundreds of people in the parks doing Tai Chi. Even in America, you see a lot of Tai Chi being practiced. It's also being used as a therapy in hospitals, particularly Tai Chi Shih, which is a simpler form, but it's still Tai Chi. My mom does Tai Chi, and she's in her late eighties. She's not going to do Push Hands or throw anybody to the ground, but a month ago she had a fall and she just rolled out of it. She said, "That was the Tai Chi." I said, "That is so awesome, Mom." She's always saying she doesn't know her form, she doesn't know what she's doing, just does it to be social. But I tell her, "Mom, that's great. Just keep doing it." Obviously she's gained benefits beyond the socializing and stuff.

There are two Tai Chi origin stories. One legend features Zhang Sanfeng, the fictional Taoist patriarch who had a vision of a crane and a snake fighting—this became the creation myth of Tai Chi. Then there's the Chen-style origin story, where the Chen family founded Chen Village and their practice. After the Cultural Revolution ended, the Chinese realized that ancient treasures like Tai Chi were actually kind of cool, and they capitalized on that. But I think the Chen masters had the greatest impact because they all went out globally and taught. They traveled the world and taught, like Master Ren.

One last thing I'd like to say: As well as being a publisher, I work for an organization called Rock Medicine as well as JMED. This is very important to me. We travel to concerts and such here in Northern California and offer basically first aid, but my focus is dealing with intense psychedelic reactions—a fancy way of saying bad drug trips. We have a number of protocols we use to help give aid. I deal with patients who need aid while under the influence. You can imagine the range of things I'm confronted with. We have worked often with bands like the Grateful Dead. I was introduced to this through martial arts. While studying for a psychology degree, I began practicing Iaido, a quick-draw sword form. My Iaido teacher was a psych tech and the founder of Rock Medicine. I have now been doing this kind of work for thirty-two years.

JON MILLER

Businessman, student of Ren GuangYi, and founder of Beckoning Path

I met Lou in 2003, at a dinner Scott arranged for me, Lou, and Ren in New York. I was looking forward to it on multiple levels, obviously. A chance to meet Lou as well as a chance to meet Master Ren. Now, I knew of Ren and had seen videos of him and was always quite impressed. And in fact, in certain ways, quite intimidated in the sense of I didn't think that I could learn that. I thought it might be a little bit too hard for me to pick up at the age of approaching fifty. A couple of things happened at that dinner. First, with regard to Master Ren, it was very clear from just some of the movements at the table that he was not only what I thought he was but even

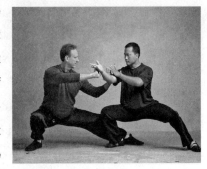

Jon Miller and Ren

something quite a bit more. It was just amazing to see, even sort of sitting down, when he would animate his conversation with points about Tai Chi. How he could illustrate them even just at the table was extraordinarily impressive to me. I remember that very vividly.

And what surprised me about Lou was, and this continued to be so in every contact we had, was not only how much he was into it but into the intricacies of it. He loved to see a little aspect of something he hadn't seen before and to kind of riff on that, and loved watching Master Ren, because he would pick up a little something. I could see that. A glimpse here, a moment there. That struck me very strongly about Lou at that dinner.

At one point, I asked Lou how he got into it and how he was able to practice. Which was really my way of saying, "Can I try this at my age?" It was his enthusiasm, and he practiced and took lessons daily. If he could do it, I could do it. It led me to start taking lessons with Master Ren the following week.

What's incredible about Master Ren is he takes real joy in his students' improvements. For Lou, you could see the joy that he would find whenever he'd find something new, how he would light up about it.

It seemed to me, whatever he was working on at that time, he was really into it and really loved to talk about that. And if you had a nuance in the form that you could show, that would animate him. I think his love of the art and love of learning the art was infectious.

With my lifestyle, I find myself on planes quite a bit. I've developed a routine on planes where I spend a bit of time literally trying to do forms or other aspects of the practice in my mind. And when you say "in the mind," it sounds abstract or unattached to your physical presence. Actually, I think when you say, "Do it in your mind," it's really with, as it's referred to, intent. And when you do it that way, it affects the body as a whole. The body-mind, as they say, as a whole.

In 2005, we sponsored an event for a conference in San Francisco, which was a tech conference. Lou was the featured attraction for the evening. It was getting reasonably late, and so, what did we do? Went back to the hotel, found a balcony, and did Tai Chi. That's what he wanted to do. We spent quite some time outside on the balcony at the hotel doing some Tai Chi together. We were comparing notes on things, we were learning. We both wanted to do that even at that hour. I remember that quite vividly and fondly.

At the Lincoln Center memorial performance for Lou in 2016, Stephan and José, who are Master Ren's two most long-standing students in the US, did a Push Hands demonstration to the song "Heroin," which is not necessarily a song one might have associated with Tai Chi, initially. And I was a little surprised by the confluence of those two things. But, in fact, I thought it was brilliant. One of the aspects of the song "Heroin," just from the musical point of view, is the pacing changes from quite slow to quite vigorous. And back and forth, Stephan and José matched the music in their demonstration of Push Hands. And Push Hands is a bridge between the more meditative aspects and the more martial aspects of the art. It has tension. It has aggression. They took these and channeled it into the art of Push Hands. Lou's music is obviously something that appeals to everybody in all cultures around the world and provides another door into the art of Tai Chi.

I think drawing those kinds of connections is important to bring people into Tai Chi. I only wish others would do more of that.

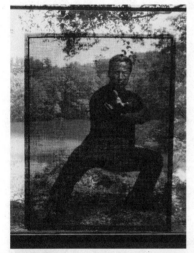

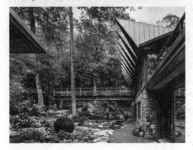

Above: Wire mesh portrait of Ren based on a photo by Lou; below: Beckoning Path in Armonk, New York

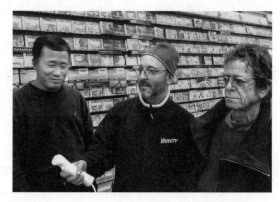

Above: Ren, Scott Richman, and Lou testing out the Nintendo Wii for possible use in interactive Tai Chi programs, 2010; below: Ren instructional video narrated by Lou and published by YMAA

EDITOR'S NOTE: SCOTT RICHMAN

In the mid- to late 2000s, Lou was taking private lessons seven days a week, three hours a day, as well as attending Master Ren's Tuesday night and Sunday morning group lessons at 440 Lafayette Street. Each class would be packed. Twenty-five-plus students jammed into a hot, sweaty five-hundred-square-foot room with beginner students spilling over into the hallway being taught by senior students like Lou. The collective mood after class, along with physical fatigue, was a high—we were happy, spirited, and our minds were bristling with ideas. Often after class, a smaller group of students including Lou and Master Ren would head over to a local restaurant to grab a meal together. We were a diverse group of students—doctors, lawyers, physicists, musicians, media, computer programmers, and athletes—who found a common passion in learning Tai Chi and studying with Master Ren.

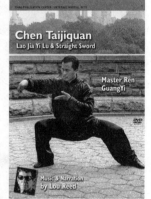

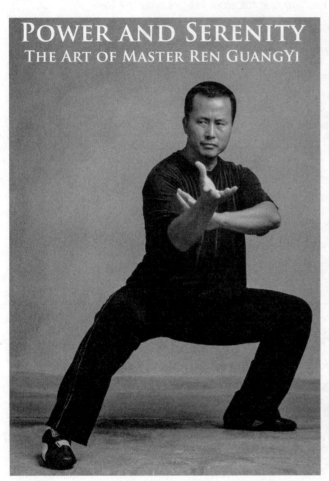

POWER AND SERENITY
THE ART OF MASTER REN GUANGYI

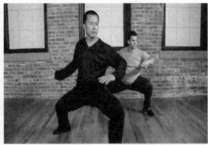

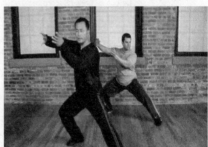

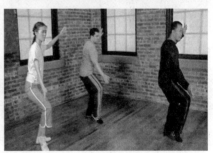

Cover (left) and stills (right) from Power and Serenity *instructional DVD, 2009*

Master Ren was always asking this smaller group to get creative and think of ways we could help promote Tai Chi and his teaching. For Lou this became something of a mission. He became the unofficial spokesperson for Chen style. At Master Ren's urging, several students, including me, would work with Lou to promote Tai Chi, creating instructional DVDs, music projects, performances, and late-night infomercials.

I remember introducing Master Ren to Jake Steinfeld of *Body by Jake*, the most popular TV health program at the time. Jake offered several ideas on how we could promote Tai Chi videos. He said we needed an exercise apparatus that we could bundle and sell with the video, like a ball or a stick. He spoke about a lot of things to Ren and me but the one big takeaway for Ren was that Ren should do a late-night infomercial so he could make money while he was sleeping. Ren never forgot that and would often ask me how we could make money while sleeping. I'm still trying to figure that out.

We also got excited when the new iPhone came out and video game platforms like the Nintendo Wii were doing physical interactive games as new exercise workouts. We contacted and met several tech and game companies to explore doing a Tai Chi–inspired game and app. Lou clearly knew that his celebrity could help Ren find a larger audience, and new technology presented a great opportunity to help find that audience. "The Art of the Straight Line" was the title Lou chose in 2009 for this book—one of the projects we set out to do to promote Tai Chi.

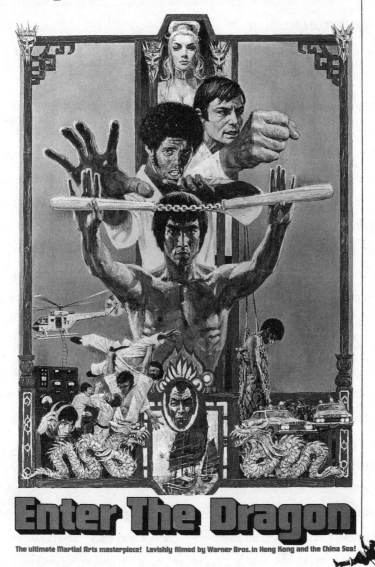

Film poster for Bruce Lee's Enter the Dragon

WARRINGTON HUDLIN

Film producer, vice-chairman of the Museum of the Moving Image, and Tai Chi practitioner

I got the opportunity to screen Stephan's film *Final Weapon* in 2011. Although I knew Stephan through the martial arts world, I did not know I was going to get all the stars of the film as part of the screening package! When Lou walked through the door, the audience was, "Oh my God, look who's here!"

The main thing I noticed about Lou was just peace. And the second thing that struck me was his curiosity. Which is also a statement of peace. Because if you're full of yourself, you can't see what's around you.

I was very impressed that the team—Lou, Ren, Stephan, José Figueroa, and the Hong Kong film legend Mike Woods—were so peaceful and calm. As a longtime film producer [*Boomerang*, *House Party*, *Bebe's Kids*, *Katrina*, *Unstoppable*], I've worked with a whole list of stars who come with entourages and disruptions. The *Final Weapon* team didn't have any of that. We had a great Q&A. And that really stood out to me. In many ways it manifested the principles of Tai Chi. Balance and harmony. Didn't disrupt. They came. They shared.

STEPHAN BERWICK: Lou was so deeply appreciative of what you did that day.

WARRINGTON HUDLIN: I was happy that he also appreciated the museum as a whole. I introduced him to the chief curator and said, "You guys, whatever you want us to do, say yes, and we should do it." They exchanged numbers.

I run two programs at the museum. One is called Changing the Picture, which is a program of films by people of color. The other is my real pleasure! I host a monthly film series called Fist and Sword, which exclusively screens martial arts movies.

STEPHAN: When you showed our piece, was that for the Fist and Sword series?

WARRINGTON: Yes. In fact, the *Final Weapon* screening was the featured event for the inauguration of the re-opening of the museum after a complete refurbishing. Recently, Michael Barker, who's co-president of Sony Pictures Classics, asked me to screen the hit Indonesian martial arts film *The Raid: Redemption* at Fist and Sword.

SCOTT RICHMAN: Lou loved *The Raid: Redemption*!

WARRINGTON: When I was young, I went to the Pagoda movie theater in Chinatown to watch martial arts movies. I watched those movies over and over. I said to my friends, "They're moving so fast. You watch the feet, I'll watch the hands. We'll figure out what they did."

I've been doing martial arts for over fifty years. I started, like many Americans, in Karate. But, as soon as I got access to Chinese martial arts, I studied with Alan Lee, who was one of the first Chinese Americans to teach non-Chinese people. Over the last decade, I discovered Tai Chi. Specifically Wu Tai Chi. I'm madly in love with it. So I can identify with Lou's passion for Tai Chi. It's a deep, deep love, because it reveals so much about yourself and the universe.

What strikes me, and my sense of kinship, if I can be bold, is if you're serious about martial arts, those things are natural. In Tai Chi, it's self-discovery. Which, by the way, is all about alignment and listening. The more you cultivate alignment with form practice, you'll hear for the first time in ways you couldn't before.

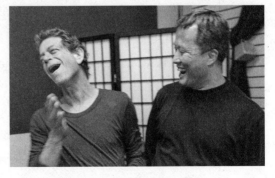

Lou and Ren on the set of Final Weapon

When I was young, I was a fighter and competed in martial arts competitions. If you think Karate is hard, and you think of Tai Chi as water, it's even more so like steam, like mist. When I do Push Hands with my teacher, he's not there. He's just not there. I can't feel him! I sometimes feel like I step into a hole in the floor. *Where was he? He was there, but he's not there.* He's like a shadow stuck to my body. I hope I have a little bit of time left to get to that. Everything is listening and making your body unify. And that's going to take me the rest of my life.

When I do Push Hands with my teacher, he's not there.

▲

MICHAEL IMPERIOLI

Actor in The Sopranos *and* Goodfellas

Lou was my hero, and seeing your hero wandering around the streets was a big deal for me. The very first time I met him was at the New York Knicks game around 1991. I told him I was playing Ondine in the film *I Shot Andy Warhol*. I knew Lou was against the movie because it was about a woman who basically almost kills one of his dear friends.

I got into martial arts in 2002. *The Sopranos* had hit, and my life really changed after that. I reached a point where I was very unhealthy—mentally and physically. I was smoking. I was drinking. I was not exercising at all. And my kids started doing Tae Kwon Do. I started studying with a teacher in Tribeca, and my wife started doing it and all my kids were doing it. The martial arts led us to Buddhism and meditation. Martial arts was a gateway for me into a spiritual path. I wouldn't doubt that that was similar for Lou. The beautiful thing is when you're doing martial arts, you can't think of anything else. There's not space in your mind to wander. There's not room for it. When you're doing something like that, your mind is completely engaged.

One of the things I really admire about Lou is that he was an artist his whole life. Like he was still discovering new things. His later albums are as good as all the albums. He's doing new material that's pushing the boundaries of rock and roll music. He managed to keep that creative spark for his whole life in a very profound way that most artists, rock and roll artists, have not been able to do. I would imagine the longevity that he had and his creativity and commitment to art, it had something to do with his Tai Chi practice.

When Lou passed away, it hit me in a very unexpected way because of what he represented to me as an artist, and his kindness and generosity towards me. It was almost the end of an era in New York and in the world.

TIMOTHY GREENFIELD-SANDERS

Photographer and filmmaker

I met Lou in '94 because of a portrait series I created for *GQ* called "Best Buddies." It was of famous people with their best friend. I thought, *Lou Reed. Who does Lou Reed hang out with?* Magician Penn Jillette at the time was the person Lou brought to the shoot.

Lou was in the closet about his Tai Chi. I knew Lou had an interest in boxing and martial arts. It was more like an interest in film, in Bruce Lee, I thought. Lou was intimate with that material. He knew everything. He saw the latest films when they came out. I wasn't particularly interested to even go with him to see those films. He would go to Canal Street in Chinatown to see them. Tai Chi was never part of my relationship with Lou until Ren.

Ren's class was a whole other world Lou had. He was very devoted. He'd come up to my country home and he'd have to go back to the city for his Sunday morning class. That's how I started to see it. When Ren became part of the scene, part of the team, and part of the environment, I started

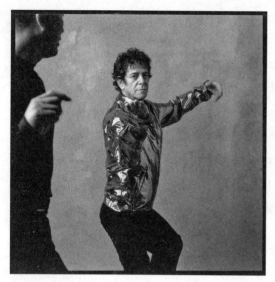

Ren directing Lou in a Timothy Greenfield-Sanders photo session

to understand the depth of Lou's commitment to it. I was invited to the classes but never went. In some ways I regret that I didn't, because it was a way to be with Lou, doing something he loved.

When I first photographed Lou in Tai Chi poses, it was extremely difficult to do, because I didn't know what the poses were. It's like photographing a dancer or musician. The Tai Chi portraits I did of Lou are probably the most loose of my portraiture, because my portraits are of the person in front of the camera being very still. I think those pictures with Ren, when they're both doing the same pose and moving through it, are fabulous.

Regardless of whether you know what is good, what the form is, you can tell there's a moment when the hand is a certain way that looks fabulous. Those were hard to shoot. They weren't Timothy Greenfield-Sanders portraits. They were something else. It was like I was capturing what was happening there, but it wasn't something I understood well.

LAURIE ANDERSON: You feel you captured it?

TIMOTHY GREENFIELD-SANDERS: I think I captured the connection between both of them very well, and even the single shots, I think, are very beautiful.

LAURIE: They had a real magnetic thing going on.

TIMOTHY: They did. They projected. I don't think Lou would have wanted to take those pictures without Ren there in some way.

SCOTT RICHMAN: You know what's interesting? The first of the photos you did with Ren and Lou was when Lou just started to work with Ren in 2002.

TIMOTHY: Oh, really? I think Ren being there allowed him to do it in his head, in a sense.

LAURIE: Why do you think that was?

TIMOTHY: Well, I think he respected Ren enormously. We all used to joke that Ren could do anything. He would take a camera, and he had a good eye. Lou liked the story of Ren too. There was a kind of mythology around Ren that was so interesting. And of course there were those tours with Ren onstage. Did the audience like it or not? Some did. Some didn't. Lou didn't care. *He* liked it.

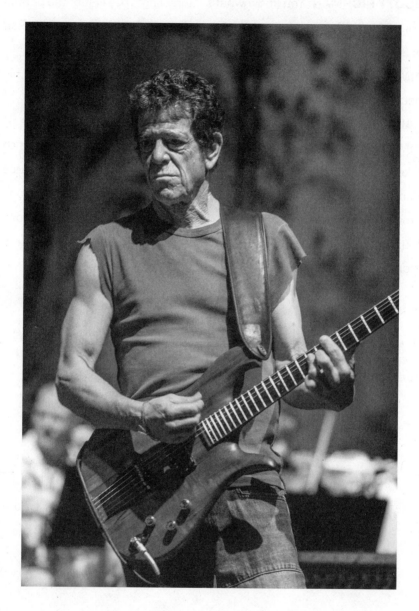

Berlin tour, London, 2008

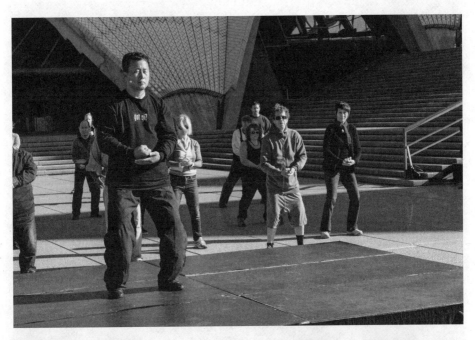

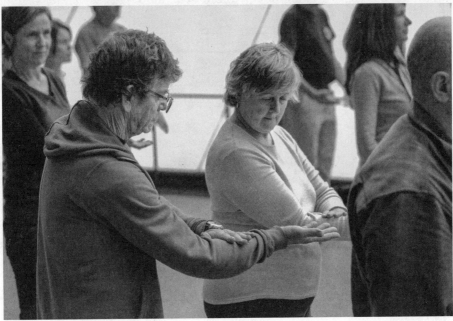

Above: Ren leading a class at the Sydney Opera House;
below: Lou teaching at the Sydney Opera House, 2010

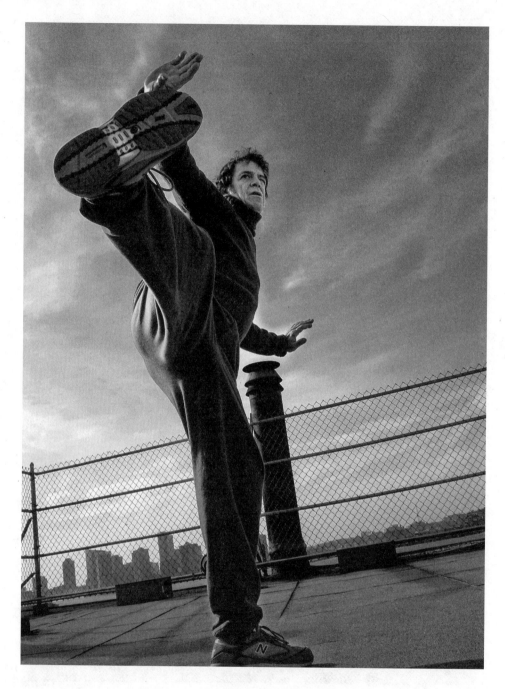

Lou practicing on the roof

CHAPTER 10

MASTERY

I accept the newfound man, and set the twilight reeling

I was swimming in the Pacific waters of Mexico—calm, serene, modest waves. I was doing my Tai Chi forms. I'd hurt my leg on a tour, and now I was trying to regain my balance and power. I was often on the tips of my toes to better help me jump. I'd been taught to try to be as fluid as possible, and what better way than a workout in the ocean. I was staring at the sun, the incomparable sunset to come. A wave broke and snatched my glasses—a gift of older age; I didn't always need them. Light in weight, they sank and waggled to a stop on the smooth ocean floor. I stood balanced in Horse pose and then one-legged stance, searching the bottom of the smooth sand, found them and plucked them up with my toes. The trade-off for not seeing and so many other physical disappointments—the rheumatoid toe, diabetes, smoking, and reckless behavior—was learning Tai Chi.

—FROM LOU'S NOTES ON TAI CHI

ROBIN GOLAND

Endocrinologist and Lou's doctor

When Lou was just becoming a patient of mine, he was struggling, as many patients do, with managing diabetes. It's such a self-care condition—taking control, managing diet, and managing the medication. One evening he called my house. Cell phones probably weren't really much used back then, and my children were small. One of my kids answered the phone and came running into the dining room, where I had a lot of people over, and yelled, "Dr. Lou Reed is on the phone." All my dinner guests went, "Oh my God, that Lou Reed?" And I went upstairs and said, "Lou, what about your confidentiality? All I do is diabetes, and you just basically announced that to the whole dinner party. And furthermore, that's not funny." He said, "Well, you're laughing." Okay, so it's a little funny. It was extremely funny. He was, as you know, extremely funny.

Even back then, he was a role model, and he was happy to talk about it. He sat in my waiting room and spoke to the children about taking their medicine and how hard it could be. He was extremely generous that way, and he took his own health very seriously—having diabetes is hard, and what we ask people to do is challenging. It's like a marathon, not a sprint, and you never get good at it, and it changes and it's difficult. It's a journey where you really do need to work with a teacher. But then the patient teaches the teacher, more than we teach them. And it was a very important and rewarding relationship over many years. Yeah, and with Lou it was fifteen years, at least.

Lou's diabetes was discovered on a blood test. So, people with hepatitis C have a higher incidence of high blood sugar for reasons that are not quite clear. And it's hard to overestimate the challenge it is to manage it. Treatment and monitoring are difficult. The management of the diet and ice cream and pancakes had been part of our discussion. But all the years I knew him, the diabetes really didn't stop him from doing anything. It was not a factor in his health, which is a tribute to the great job he did in keeping himself healthy.

His relationship with me went in both directions, and I miss him. I know that's frivolous to say, but people who had the privilege to take care of him all felt that way.

One last thing: Back to ice cream and pancakes—for him and many patients, the problem is the "once in a while" problem. He and I had a long discussion about ice cream. He loved ice cream. I said, "Really, it's my job to help you have any food that you want. But the key is moderation." And we agreed that every now and again, one small scoop of ice cream would be fine and perfectly compatible with good glucose control. This again was pre–cell phone because my children remember this conversation. He called me up and told me he was going to do it. And I told him, "Go for it. It's not going to hurt you. You'll be perfectly fine. And don't even check your blood sugar, because it'll be a little high, but it will come down and it won't hurt you. It's a once-every-month treat." He called me later and he said, "It was really good, so I had three scoops." I said, "Okay, that's not such a good idea." Then of course the discussion was, "Well, this was your fault. You should have been able to see this coming. Who eats half a scoop of ice cream?" He was a wonderful man.

YAMUNA

Bodywork practitioner who treated Lou

It was 2003 or 2004 when Lou just walked by and came in. After that, he would come by occasionally. When my husband died, I was sick of being in town. I just didn't want to be around. It was too painful. Lou had started coming to the studio by then. First, he took classes, and then he came all the time. I remember he came to a class about his feet when he had plantar fasciitis, and there were about fifty people in this class. Most people forget what I say, but he paid attention, he got it, and he fixed one foot, then the other. He could fix himself. When I said too much, he teased me. "Just shut up and tell me what I need to do. Make it clear."

He had something that I've never seen in anyone. Never. It was really something, and calling it "vital force" is a really great way to comprehend it—he paid attention and tried to do things.

And Lou always had something to say. He was already doing Tai Chi a long time before we met. He came in one day and said, "You know I could kill you with one move, if I had a sword in my hand right now." And I'd say, "Okay, Lou, that's really good. I'm glad you're that strong." Or he might talk about taking care of my dogs. He had the same kind, dachshunds. He'd yell, "I had one of those. You've got to watch the hips. Take care of the hips. Don't let him jump." Or he'd say things like, "Why do women in the neighborhood hate you?" But I just kept working on him.

Then he thought I was a bad businessperson because I didn't want to see him three times a week. I said, "That's overload. You're already working with Ren every day, and you're doing all this work on yourself." I think he respected me for that, because I said, "Look, I don't want to just take your money." Also, he had ideas for stuff related to the studio, techniques and products, and Lou would say, "How do you think people are going to know what you do?"

He had an amazing body to work on and he had a very smart body. A smart body means a body that can take information in quickly. I have my own way of measuring energy and how strong pulses are, and Lou's vital force was always on, except when he was taking interferon, the drug for his liver disease. Then I would feel his pulse and know there was nothing to work with. "They're killing me. What am I supposed to do?" I couldn't work on him and said, "You're too weak. Your body is too weak."

He couldn't work with swords at all. He was too weak and would say to me, "So when do you think I'll be able to do it?" and I would have to say, "Look, I know you're on this drug. I know it's for a certain amount of time,

A smart body means a body that can take information in quickly.

▲

and I think that your body's not accepting this, but I'm not a doctor. I just know you." He was just getting lower and lower and lower. I said to him, "After you get off this, give yourself six months, go easy and just build your body back. Don't push yourself. Trust Ren and just slowly build up. Don't do too much because you're really debilitated and you'll get injured." Of course after getting off the interferon he would come to me with inju-

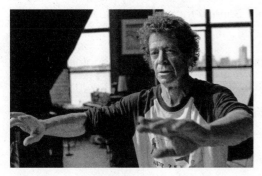

Lou training at home

ries. He would say, "Look, I can't drink, I can't do drugs, I can't smoke. There's not a whole lot of fun enjoyments out there. I can't do the things I used to like, so I now have to eat healthy."

His body was actually organized and corrected itself very quickly. And that was why I believed that his vital force was going to keep going. I really believed that even with the diabetes, which always puts a damper on everything.

Another thing I want to say about Lou is he felt energy. Lou understood energy. When someone understands energy, there are no words for it. He understood what I was doing, and he was a friend.

DANIEL RICHMAN

Pain management doctor at the Hospital for Special Surgery in New York City and Tai Chi student

One of my patients was studying with Master Ren. He is an accomplished Tai Chi student and has won many martial arts competitions. I'd asked him, "You know, your back is horrible. How is it your legs are so strong?" And he said, "Tai Chi." I asked, "What's Tai Chi?" And he explained it to me a little bit.

I had hurt my neck. I had a support collar on, and he said, "You should be doing Tai Chi." And I said, "Oh, I don't want to do martial arts. I'm in so much pain right now. I can't." He said, "You have to study with my teacher. He's the best." I said, "Who is your teacher?" And he said, "Ren GuangYi." I asked, "Is he the one that tours with Lou Reed?" He says, "Yeah." "I just met him," I told him. "Well, that's where you have to go, to his class." I went a week later on a Sunday morning on Lafayette Street. It was early March of 2004.

I had only been doing Tai Chi for six or seven weeks and my doctor and friend Seth Waldman looked at me and said, "This doesn't help your pain, does it?" And I said, "You know, I hadn't even thought about it." And he said, "Well, how's your pain?" And I said, "It's not that bad." And that was the very beginning. That was sort of the first glimmer, when I felt like, *Wow, either this is a spontaneous resolution or this is real.*

I guess another three or four months go by, and Ren offers me private lessons. So I was doing a class once a week and a lesson once a week, and I was in exercise-posture heaven. The pain was getting better. Everything was getting better. My life was getting better in every way. I met Lou at that time, and I realized he was very intense about his studying Tai Chi. He was doing lessons every day—seven days a week. He was learning something new every day. He was having, I would say, light bulbs going off as to how to do certain things and what it meant and how it felt. The way he would say, you know, a millimeter this way or that. It's intense strength, power, if your hand is this way or that way. And all of that was just very helpful from Lou. I just looked up to him as a mentor. In the time that I knew Lou, I not only learned from him and practiced with him but I also treated him as a patient.

During class, I'm in the corner learning with the beginners. I'm looking at people, but I don't understand what they're doing yet. I can't believe I'm going to get to that point. Lou would teach me, and he would always stress the idea of patience and not going too fast. When Ren would show you a form, he breaks it up. If you try to go to the next spot and he hasn't okayed you to go to the next spot, it's like, "Oh, you're not ready for that." This is what makes Ren so special. He understands, like all great teachers. They're seeing what their students take in, what they're learning, and they're not pushing them to it. Because, you know, if you're a teacher and you push your student too hard, they'll quit. It's one of those things where you cannot compare it to something like running or cycling, where you let your mind go free. Tai Chi doesn't do that. I find that Tai Chi actually allows me to focus. When I put my whole mind and heart into it, I get so much more out of it. I say, *Okay, where am I? Is my hand here? Am I feeling . . . What am I feeling?* So that next time I come around to this part I can remember to do it this way, or I think about what Ren taught me. So I am thinking about it, but I am also trying to empty my mind of any negativity. I don't have to try. It just happens.

Watching Lou touring, it was less than glamorous. Hotels, the buses, the this, the that, and I have to say, one of the reasons I believe Lou liked having Master Ren, Scott, or me, or any of his Tai Chi buddies, on tour was that it took him away from the rock and roll celebrity world, from being a band leader when he wasn't onstage, and that responsibility. It was a helpful stress reliever. He would do Tai Chi to help relax, get focused. I think it helped him be more effective in what he was doing. It seemed to me that on a rock and roll tour the only really good time is when you're doing a show. You're out there performing, and you've got a good crowd. Your band is right, and the sound is right. So all that other stuff in between, if you can make it a little bit better with Tai Chi and doing it at a high level, then that was a bonus for Lou.

The first time I noticed the energy thing was probably the fourth or fifth private lesson I had at Master Ren's house. I had just started the core Chen Tai Chi training form Lao Jia Yi Lu [Old Frame First Road], and he was showing me another form, the more fundamental 38 Movement Form. I said, "No, I already know this." And he says, "No, no. You've got to know it the private lesson way, you know, corrections and the whole thing." He did a one-hour 38 with me—he was doing it with me.

In the beginning, in privates, he does it with you. It's not like him watching, because you don't know what you're doing yet as far as he's concerned. So he's got to stop, and I could see in his eyes this energy, as if he had ten cups of coffee without any of the negativity about that. I was like, "Oh my God." Instead of being tired, he just took me through this hour of intensity. And I said, "Not only don't I have any pain right now, not only am I not tired, I feel this boost of energy as if I was being replenished." It was like I was feeling this redemption of energy. I told Lou, and he said, "Now you've got it."

ELINOR GREENBERG

Private student of Ren GuangYi and leading New York psychologist

I'm a psychologist, working as a psychotherapist for forty-plus years, and I always wanted a Tai Chi practice. When I was in my late twenties I had a dozen Tai Chi lessons and I loved it. I found it transformative, because I was so angry at the time, and when my hands went over my head, my anger shifted to something more neutral in that particular movement. I never forgot that. Many years later, I tried Tai Chi at health spas, but those were spas. I tried different teachers, all without success.

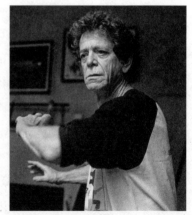

Lou training at home

In 2007, I had minor sciatica surgery for a back injury but suffered increasing pain and distress. I eventually went to Ren's student, the pain specialist Dr. Dan Richman. After he treated me, I asked, "What else can I do?" I felt very vulnerable and frail. Dan gets into an extremely low Tai Chi pose—very grand, in his white jacket, in front of the medical staff—and says, "You can do as I do, you can study with Master Ren. But he's Tai Chi master to the stars. He's very busy and is out on the road with Lou Reed." This was the first I heard of that. Dan then said, "Master Ren doesn't speak a lot of English, but you will have no trouble understanding him, because he'll read your energy. When you see him in person, you'll have no problem."

Dan said he went to the park with Ren in the morning and I could go there to meet him. I'm not a morning person, but he said it would be easier then. He would facilitate our meeting. There was no language barrier because I was injured, and Ren would just look at me and say, "You want some water?" Or he'd stop in the midst of something to tell me a story. I understood this was great politeness on his part. I was frightened, because I still had sciatica. Plus I was very bad at choreography, so I had to reassure Ren that I would learn eventually.

At that time, he did not give me hands-on corrections. Then one week I saw two doctors, and none of them had been able to help me. My sacrum was out of alignment, which happened a lot from falling, and there was nothing they did that helped. Ren said, "If you don't mind, I do this for Lou sometimes. Maybe I try for you?" He adjusted me in Zhan Zhuang ["standing like a post"] until the pain went away. It was astounding to me. It was like magic. The idea that perfect position could take away pain, a light bulb lit up. He did it a couple of times and asked me to walk. I lost it while I was walking, so we went back to adjusting, and again he brought me back. The corrections were so small, and for

The idea that perfect position could take away pain, a light bulb lit up.

▲

years, whenever Ren would do anything to me, he would first tell me, "I *Getting rid* do this for Lou." When Lou had his heel pain, I had my knee pain, and *of anger* Ren would bring me the medicine. He said, "I gave this to Lou. It helps *was one* him a lot." This was my introduction to Lou before I met him. *of the first*

I trained privately with Ren twice per week but was interested *things I* in going to a group class. The first time I did was at the 2007 Chen *remember* Xiaowang seminar in Flushing, with Lou and Stephan in front of me. *Ren talked* At the workshop, Ren points out Lou and says he was just part of the *about.* group at that point. I was more fixated on Stephan's form. But Lou made himself just part of the group, and it was so interesting to me, in ▲ light of later meetings, how he managed his energy.

I had of course heard Ren talk about Chen Xiaowang. One of the things he said about his teacher stuck with me because it was about anger. Getting rid of anger was one of the first things I remember Ren talked about—that Chen Xiaowang never gets angry. Ren told me about his own history and how he had been angry and fought in the streets.

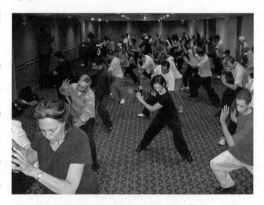

When I needed a solution to some teenage boys hanging out on my townhouse stoop, what does the martial arts master tell me to do? I had a German shepherd guard dog at the time—Jenna. I thought that was the solution. I'd come down with Jenna, *Chen Xiaowang seminar in Flushing, Queens, mid-2000s* everybody leaves. But no. Ren said, "When you water your plants, make sure the stoop gets good and wet. Use your Tai Chi." So I've been using that ever since, because it works really well. Nobody wants to sit on a wet stoop. I don't have to explain myself. I don't have to threaten them.

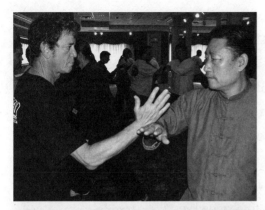

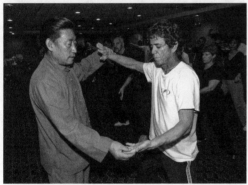

Chen Xiaowang seminar in Flushing, Queens, mid-2000s

I'm an Ericksonian hypnotherapist, which teaches how to observe, because you have someone in trance. Ericksonian approaches taught me the micro-observances of color changes, tiny muscular relaxation, and establishing an idiopathic response ahead of time for people who don't want to move. When I use Tai Chi with some of my clients, it has to come from an angle of surprise. I had a number of people I used Tai Chi with, because they had no preparation for it. They didn't have a story about what I was going to do. I used the principle from Erickson to use what you've got.

[Editors' Note: Elinor hypnotized those present in the room when she was interviewed for the book.]

Ren of course can manage his energy to be soft or hard, but I noticed Lou could manage his energy in the same fashion, which fascinated me. I'm struck by the lineage to Lou. It takes three generations, I was told, to make a lady. You have to start with her grandmother. Chen Xiaowang is the grandfather, Ren is the father, Lou is the son.

I next saw Lou at an event Dan organized at the Hospital for Special Surgery in New York City. Freddie Gershon—also a patient of Dan's, whom he referred to Ren—and I attended. I knew that Dan organized it to acquaint the doctors with the benefits of Tai Chi for patients and to raise funds. I was there early and heard two presentations before the one that

Lou and Dan gave on how to get more wealthy patients to the hospital. It's true, we were also the most injured. Rich and injured. I watched Lou's energy change at the event. He was in a T-shirt, while everyone else wore suits or doctor uniforms. But when he got to the podium, he showed total control and charisma without hesitation, speaking to the group. It was early in the morning, and he was fresh, with a warm glow. I don't remember most of what he said except the command he took. He didn't do rock star defiant, he did serious. Lou said, "This is an important thing I'm going to tell you. Listen to it because it's going to change lives."

EDDIE STERN

Yoga teacher, author, worked with Lou

I do Ashtanga Yoga, which is a very difficult kind of Yoga. I also teach Yoga therapy and adaptive things. If a person invites me to teach, I assume they actually want to do Yoga. What that means is they are interested in their soul. They're interested in the essence of their being, because you don't come to Yoga just for back pain. You don't come to it because your feet hurt or even if you have high blood pressure. You come to it because you're interested in the essential core of your being. And because you hear this word "Yoga," you have an idea that maybe it might help you tap into that. If people have problems, I work with ways to get around those problems and help make them better, the best I can.

I first met Lou at a 2006 birthday party for one of my students, Julian Schnabel. I sat next to Laurie and my wife next to Lou. I had first impressions of Lou already because I grew up on MacDougal Street during the '90s. I always say I was weaned at the Sunday hardcore matinees at CBGBs. I used to see Lou walking around the West Village, especially

West 4th Street, all the time. There was always someone yelling, "Hey, Lou," and he would wave back. I think that's cool. I never yelled it to him, but it's definitely a visual memory. By the time I met Lou, he was an icon to me. But when I first met him, I was really struck by how grumpy he was.

The second time was at his *Berlin* show at St. Ann's Warehouse. Julian invited me. Afterwards he brought us backstage and said to Lou, "This is my Yoga teacher. You should do some Yoga with him." Lou replied, "I hate Yoga. It hurts my knees." I just thought that was so funny. That's not normally a first response to get from someone you've never met before. I thought that was just really funny and unfiltered and I liked it. I also took it as a challenge because I thought, *Here's someone who hates Yoga, but maybe they don't know what I do.*

I first taught him in 2007. I was nervous going into our first class because I thought, *What am I going to do with this guy?* When I first came in, Lou told me everything that was wrong with him and everything that he couldn't do. So that limited the amount of things that I could do. We did really simple things, including stretches, breathing, and a bit of meditation. At the end, he was very happy and gave me a warm handshake and hug. He said, "That was great. Let's do it again." I thought that was wonderful.

And every time he would tell me exactly what he wanted to do that day because he was doing Tai Chi all week. He said, "I'm doing six days a week of Tai Chi. I'm going to do one day a week of Yoga. So this one day is where I'm gonna fill in the other stuff." He'd say, "So today, stretching and meditation." Or, "Today, I need to do breathing. I'm really tired. I just wanna lie down, and maybe you can do that thing you did on my neck or something." I would try my best to do it.

His knees were always a problem, so he always wanted to do something about that. We'd always do a lot of hip things to strengthen the

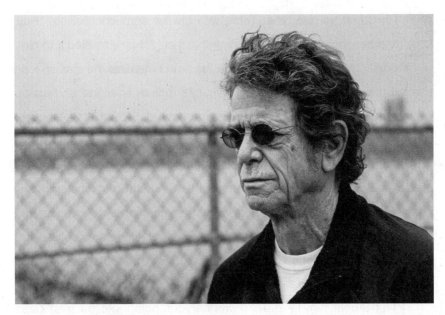

Lou on his roof overlooking the Hudson River

quadriceps. Although, his were fairly good from all the Tai Chi he did. But his feet were not always at the top of the menu. They were definitely things we worked on, and sometimes I would just give him a foot massage and do things for his arches and ankles.

We talked about Yoga and Tai Chi in regard to energy. For me, Yoga postures are only peripheral and are a way to access the nervous system and the mind. Most of the poses and all of the breathing practices are for purification of the nervous system. And the nervous system is how we organize our physiology with the outer environment we live in. Tai Chi is the same thing. You're pulling yourself into different flows with the external environment through the movements. It's merging our mind through the nervous system and through the body into our extended body, which is the world around us.

That was very easy to access with Lou and Yoga, because he had that internal understanding from Tai Chi. We talked about that. We didn't talk about strengthening core muscles, for example. We talked about an-atomical things sometimes, but the main thing he wanted was to calm his mind and be clear and relaxed by the time he was done.

Sometimes he'd pick up a sword and demonstrate Tai Chi, saying, "This move hurts my shoulder here. What can I do?" And then we would do shoulder stretches or shoulder strengthening or I'd do something to counterbalance that particular move, so he could do it without pain. That was fun too. He would do that probably every third or fourth lesson. Every system, when it's repetitive, has a drawback. Every system has a flaw. Yoga as well, very much so. Sometimes you can pick things from other systems to stop the repetitive nature of something else. That's one of the ways we tried to use the practice for him. As the body ages, it can't take the thrusting and heavy weight of weapons. I didn't know how he handled some of those things! I was amazed.

We also talked a lot about new exercise machines he tried. I think the only things that really seemed to work for Lou were Tai Chi and Yoga. Those were the only consistent things. When we talked about Yoga, we discussed philosophy, Tai Chi, and physical things. For example, he once wanted to get six-pack abs. He wanted to have a tight belly. I thought, *I don't have that! I don't even know if I can train him to do that. I can train him to be strong.*

SCOTT RICHMAN: Which relates to the tour diary he wrote in 1996 in *The New Yorker*, about Iggy Pop. He wrote, "I'm doing crunches every day because I'd like to have six-pack abs like Iggy."

EDDIE STERN: Lou would always say, "I have this friend, Rick Owens [the fashion designer], who goes to the gym two hours a day and he's completely ripped. Can I get like that from Yoga?"

We also talked about recovery. I think there are certain themes that are im-portant for anyone who's in recovery, like gratitude, appreciation, forgiveness, letting go, and surrender. I think these are the five major things that any human being needs to work on. In recovery, those are important. We talked about those things a lot. Lou would get angry very quickly about things. He didn't want to have that kind of reactive mind. He wanted to conquer his anger, and that's one of the things we talked about regarding Yoga and meditation.

Doing things like Yoga, breathing, and meditation can help calm the nervous system. But there's always the pattern we have wired into us and it's beyond the nervous system. We don't know where it comes from, when something doesn't go our way and we react. For Lou, sometimes that was anger. In our conversations, he was aware of that and he wanted to get over it. We talked about our experiences of what it felt like to get angry. What it felt like to lose control and feel bad about it afterwards. Those types of conversations were as integral to the Yoga we did, because Yoga is supposed to move us to a self-reflective, self-aware state of mind to deal with our sense of humanity.

Lou was such a genuine human being. And I felt that he was so loving and caring in all of our interactions. When he would greet me, it was so warm. When I left and he was happy with the class, it was so genuine. But then sometimes I would hear him on the phone yelling at the telecoms person, and I would just sit and wait for the storm to pass.

Even if you read in books about Zen masters, you always read about how it's okay to have strong emotions as long as you don't kill or beat up someone. Things can pass over you. You can have a strong emotion and then it can just pass away like a cloud. Lou didn't seem to hold on to those things for a long time, at least what I observed. He apologized before reacting when he got angry. I appreciated and liked that.

He would express gratitude for his practices and his teachers. He would express a lot of gratitude and appreciation for the Tai Chi community that he really valued. Anytime he would reflect on or talk about his Tai Chi teacher or the community or his Buddhist teacher, automatically he would express appreciation for having them in his life. And that he was appreciative to be around these kinds of people. It made him happy. His gratitude just flowed from him naturally.

He didn't talk much about his illness with me. He was never descriptive or shared details of it. He would just say, "My liver really hurts." And then we would breathe, meditate, or chant. The techniques that helped most were the ones that helped him relax so he could sleep for a little while. When he was still well enough to do postures, we would do a few stretches. We would then do a little meditation, then sleep. Towards the last few months of our classes together, that's what we were going for. As he got more sick, we just did meditation. And I would give him some massages usually on the neck, shoulders, or feet. Meditation was not very long because after a few minutes he would start talking or he would say that something hurt. When it went well, he would fall asleep. I thought that was good. Whenever he fell asleep like that, I would let him sleep, and I would stay there until he woke up. And he was very gentle, fragile, and very open.

He would play the Tai Chi music he wrote. It was *Hudson River Wind Meditations*, an exquisite piece of music he'd play during every class we had. And we'd talk about how he didn't even know how he made those sounds and how he didn't think he could re-create them if he tried.

LAURIE ANDERSON: He didn't actually grasp the "I know why." I think that was part of his structure of how to make things. We talked about it a lot. That lack of confidence and "wow" is what keeps you from making the next thing. And makes you think, *Oh, that wasn't even what I was trying to do, that didn't even work.* He didn't think that stuff worked very well.

EDDIE: I think both of you are perfectionists. And the good thing about a perfectionist is that they're never satisfied with anything they do, which always spurs them on to be more creative.

LAURIE: The sad thing is that they think their own work is just nothing important or interesting to other people.

EDDIE: I read something that you wrote, about the three rules for living that you and Lou had. Number one, to not be afraid of anyone. Number two, always have your bullshit detector on. And number three, be as tender as possible. I love that so much. When I travel the world, teaching workshops and giving lectures, I talk about those rules and say, "These are Lou and Laurie's three rules for living, and I think there's nothing in Yoga that parallels these rules. You don't have to learn any Sanskrit. You don't have to stand on your head. If you can do these three things, I think you could live a happy life."

LAURIE: That's what we hope this book does. To get some of that spirit of "Here's something this guy learned during his life. You can learn it too."

CHARLIE MILLER

Lou's transplant surgeon

I met Lou probably six months before the transplant. I wondered how his life had changed over time. How it changed from the '60s to then. How he maintained his life. It appears that mostly his problem came from early drug use. He hadn't been using drugs for years—what had he been doing to take care of himself? I discovered he was compulsive and precise about taking care of himself. But people have a bias particularly about transplants. He had hep C. He got it from drugs. So is he still doing drugs? No, he's doing Tai Chi. We shouldn't judge so fast.

Lou, though, was sick as hell and was getting sicker. He knew he was dying. We were just hoping for a second shelf liver. We didn't know when we would get one, so he was constantly flying to and from Cleveland for treatment. You can't imagine what that kind of uncertainty does to the soul. But he had this inner strength. He needed a liver, and when we found one, there was no hesitation. "We're doing it," he said. I was totally candid about the circumstances and the less-than-perfect liver. Two thousand people turned it down. It was not good enough for most people, but he said, "Well, it's good enough for me. Let's go." He was a very good advocate for himself.

Lou could go from laughing to crying, being angry and cursing to smiling and telling a joke in a matter of seconds, but he remained centered. You only needed to tell him something once, and what we were telling him was very complicated. He got it in the snap of your fingers.

The surgery went well, and he was up and doing his thing in a couple of days. I could see Lou's calm and strength. Maybe it was spiritual. He was centered—his spirit was centered. He had a core spiritual and physical strength as a result, I think, of doing Tai Chi.

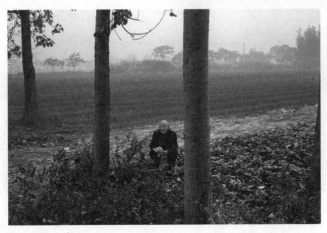

Photo of an elderly person taken by Lou in Chen Village

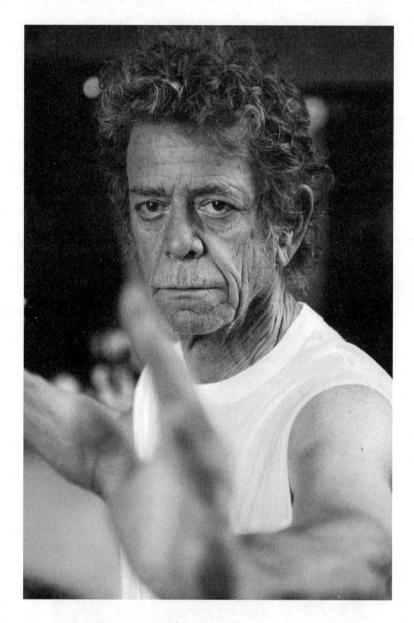

Lou on guard

BOB CURRIE

Editor

My relationship with Lou was a simple thing. It was simply friendship. I didn't work with him or for him; it was just the luck of getting to know someone and ending up with an amazing friend. And he was that, a true and kind friend to so many. That's really the whole story.

We met in 2006 or 2007, at Bouley's Café. We had dinner upstairs, Laurie, Lou, poet Anne Carson, and me. Pretty quickly, we just started hanging out. Those days usually began with breakfast at Café Cluny or somewhere else in the West Village and went from there. He would invariably be late, which gave me time to read or do a bit of writing. Lou would show up, we'd eat and talk about everyday stuff, what he should get Shirley for her birthday or what Laurie was doing on the road. So it was just that friendship, at least for me. It could potentially go on for hours, but the cutoff was seeing Ren. "I'm going to do Tai Chi."

Like we've asked everyone for this book, "Did he ever talk about Tai Chi and did he ever try to get you to do it?" and of course the answer to both is yes. After a couple of months, he said, "You should try this out," and I think the first time I did anything with Tai Chi was going over to the apartment on 11th Street, when Ren was there. It was, *Wow, I get a free lesson.*

An early memory of Ren was maybe the second time I met him, and he had us doing Standing Mountain, Master Ren's name for standing post training. He came over and adjusted two fingers on my right hand. It just shot energy through my whole body. It was extraordinary. And first, I thought, *This guy is amazing*, and the second thought was, *I want to always do it wrong, so he'll fix it, so I get that feeling again*. It was such a powerful thing.

Lou was right, and though I'm not very good at it, and don't practice enough, it did change everything. There's a calmness and an openness that came from doing Tai Chi.

Anne Waldman talked about Lou being a poet and his love of poetry, so it was not surprising, if Lou was in town and Anne Carson was reading somewhere, he would be there. And if I said, "Lou, there's this really interesting reading going on," he would be there. He was always ready to go out and hear someone read some poetry or fiction.

Like those other ten thousand people, I bought that Velvets first album in the '60s. At the time, I was listening to contemporary classical music, like John Cage or free jazz like Ornette Coleman or the Art

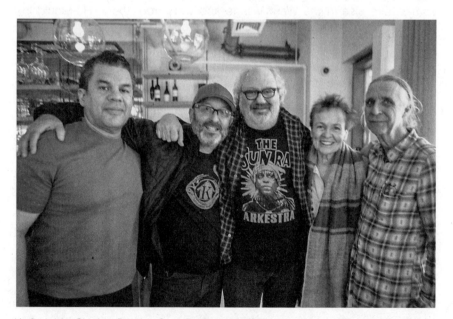

Left to right: Stephan Berwick, Scott Richman, Hal Willner, Laurie Anderson, and Bob Currie

Ensemble of Chicago, and when I heard that record, not knowing Lou was responsible for it, it made me realize that you could actually tell a complete story in a song. I hadn't known that before. It was just that ability to use a minimal amount of language, work from a small detail, to create a maximum kind of story. Maybe Smokey Robinson, occasionally, could pull it off, you know, with "Tears of a Clown" or some others, but what Lou did was just profound. It was a different way of using language as lyric. It was just exciting to listen to that record. After the Velvets, I continued to listen to Lou. I loved *Metal Machine Music*. Years later, it was so cool to be at the rehearsals of Metal Machine Trio.

When Lou started taking interferon, Laurie had to tour a lot, and she'd give me a call, and I would come back to the city from wherever we were and spend time with him. Breakfast, lunch, dinner, and more. I was lucky, I had the time to do it. There are a dozen people who would've done that if they had the time, so that bit's nothing special. He was somebody I loved, and it was wonderful to be part of his life.

We were sitting at Sant Ambroeus when Lou got a call from the doctor. He said the interferon hadn't worked. Lou hung up and simply said, "What are you having for breakfast?" I was shocked at the calmness in that moment. You have to remember how horrible that drug is. It rages and creates weird cognitive stuff, weird everything, and terrible emotional pain and an irrational anger. Everything was emotionally and physically charged. It would be the whole range all the time. He was so vulnerable. But he managed to talk about it. It was the same after the transplant. He talked mostly with Kevin Hearn about being sick. Kev understood it all and was incredibly kind. What he and I talked more about was the next step of getting well or lunch or Laurie. We all had different roles on the Lou healthcare spreadsheet—which was a real thing.

People have talked about the anger he carried, and of course it was real and we all saw it, but he was a sweet and tender person, and one of the smartest and most perceptive people one could meet. You couldn't just slide things past him. Lou considered everything and then was fearless in decisions or opinions. And anyone who knew him can remember the feeling when you got the laugh or that slight upturn of a smile.

The last time I saw Lou was at the Cleveland Clinic the Thursday before he passed away. Seeing him through the open doors of the ambulance taking him to the airport and back to the Springs (in the Hamptons), it felt like goodbye.

Through the summer after the transplant, there were repeated hospital stays, but all was marked by his extraordinary strength, determination, and tireless research—his amazing will. The last night, his final night in Cleveland, it was Wednesday. Lou just started talking in that most joyful and fantastical way he had. Full of pleasure, humor, and imagination. It was thrilling. I don't remember the story, but it is thanks to Lou, that is how I will always remember him.

SCOTT RICHMAN

Collaborator and fellow Tai Chi practitioner

My brother, Danny, introduced me to Lou's music when I was in high school in 1984. He told me to buy *Rock 'n' Roll Animal*—which I did and listened to nonstop. A few days later, I went to the record store and bought his new record, *New Sensations*. How was this even the same person on each of these two records? Everything seemed different. His voice, the guitars—it had to be two different people. For me, it was first all about the lyrics, the

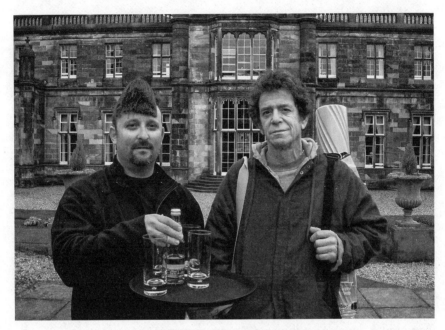

Scott and Lou in Scotland, 2005

words to the songs that drew me in; the subject matter could be both harsh and challenging, and sweet and tender. That was Lou.

Everything changed from that moment. I started to explore all of his music and writing, and the extensions and natural offshoots—the beat writers, punk and indie college, alternative rock and experimental music, poetry and journalism. Like many, I soon realized that Lou's work with the Velvet Underground from 1964 to 1970 set the course for what became modern alternative, noise, punk, industrial, and heavy metal music styles. Hal Willner used to often say that Lou was as important to rock as Miles Davis was to jazz.

Fast-forward eighteen years: I was working at AOL Music, and Lou was working on his new record, *The Raven*, with AOL's sister company Warner Bros. Records. Through Timothy Greenfield-Sanders and Annie

Ohayon (whom I'd worked with ten years earlier at Arista), I was introduced to Lou based on my interest in helping him promote *The Raven* to our large music audience. I'd met Lou a few times over the years since college, but this was a formal "sit down" meeting where we met for lunch at Pastis in the West Village. We ate, chain-smoked, and talked nonstop for three hours that day about his music, the new record, and his work. He was very open, unguarded, and unfiltered, which I really appreciated. He asked me what it was like working for Assholes On Line (AOL). He never minced words. It was also Yom Kippur 2002. How apropos to feast on the only day that the Jewish religion required us to fast to atone for our sins? I left the lunch that day thinking I would reconnect with him in a few weeks so I could get plans together. He called me the next day, eager to get into everything. If Lou trusted you, you were all in and he relied on you. That was the start of a wonderful friendship for the next eleven years, until he passed.

We talked and worked on projects in music, movies, tours, books, and of course his deep interest in the martial arts. Lou introduced me to Master Ren and took me to class with him. That was also the start of a great friendship and relationship that I have with Master Ren. With no martial arts background, it was incredibly challenging to learn Tai Chi and study with Master Ren. Master Ren is one of the best teachers I have ever had at anything, and here I was studying with him alongside Lou and other students. As Lou would say, everything he studied up until meeting Ren in 2001 paled in comparison. He said, "Ren is the real deal—no joke." Lou was always afraid of losing Ren since he was worried that Ren would leave the US and go back to China because he couldn't earn enough money teaching here. I enjoyed watching the relationship between them grow strong over those eleven years. To me, it appeared to be a brotherly type of relationship—but one that could get quite intense. Two very strong personalities coming together, sparks could fly indeed. I sometimes acted as the mediator and peacekeeper between the two. I know Stephan Berwick served that role too. However, I observed a great amount of love and respect that they each had for the other.

One of the many projects we worked on was a DVD in 2006 called *Power and Serenity: The Art of Master Ren GuangYi.* We created a new instruction and demonstration video for Silk Reeling, the 19 Form, and other streaming videos for the 21 Form and Compact Cannon Fist. Lou and Sarth Calhoun would create seven new instrumental songs to accompany the video, and fellow students Tony Visconti, Hsia-Jung Chang, Dan Richman, and Stephan would accompany Master Ren. A true Tai Chi family affair.

Hal Willner used to affectionately refer to us as the Tai Chi mishpucha.

▲

Lou knew so much about so many things in life—people, politics, art, of course music, and gear of all kinds. If you ever were thinking about buying a new camera, watch, automobile, pair of shoes, you could rely on Lou to have investigated and researched everything so thoroughly. He was like a recommendation engine. The Lou that I knew, and the Lou that many of our interviewees shared here in the book, was a complex, passionate, and ever-evolving person. In music, poetry, photography, and ultimately the martial arts, he always challenged himself first. And if his audience came aboard, well, that was great too. He knew that the martial arts, and specifically Tai Chi, was a course of study that would never have an end point. He would always be learning as well as teaching what he learned to me and others. Incredible generosity. Hal Willner used to affectionately refer to us as the Tai Chi mishpucha (Yiddish for "family").

Lou would like it when we came to visit him in the Springs, when he and Laurie bought their home in 2009. Around 2011, he was taking some new medications for his liver, and he would often be in incredible pain, with legs jumping, and I recall the image of Lou hitting his thigh to help manage the pain. Other times he was serene. Pain had subsided and he was free. I recall one visit where Master Ren and I visited Lou and Laurie, and Lou was taking new medication and couldn't drive. Lou enjoyed driving in his convertible to the beach or East Hampton with his new border terrier, Willie, running along the side of the car. He was happy we were there, but I could tell he was frustrated that he couldn't show us around on his own. In July 2012, my brother, Danny, and I drove out to the Springs to practice Tai Chi and attend Robert Wilson's Watermill Center gala on a rainy Saturday night with Lou, along with Ralph Gibson and his wife, Mary Jane. On Sunday, my brother went back to Hampton Bays, and Lou and I spent time cleaning up around the house, swimming in the saltwater pool, and doing Tai Chi. We decided later in the day—even though it was still raining—to go to Louse Point to swim.

Lou loved the water, and Louse Point, which was close to his home, was one of Lou's favorite places to swim and hang out. We waded into the water even though we saw sharp flashes of lightning farther off in the sound. We were determined to swim in the water before we headed back later that night to the city. Little Will was on a leash and Lou and I were bobbing in the water when the rain just opened up and we were slammed with heavy drops of water hitting our heads. We both lowered our chests and heads into the water halfway to where our mouths were covered and our eyes were at sea level as the rain pelted the water. We looked on in amazement as it appeared the water was coming from the bay and falling up—an optical illusion with a dark gray sky flashing in the background, but for a short time, maybe two minutes, I felt like the earth was spinning in the opposite direction. It was a moment that I will never forget, and he and I talked about it for the rest of the day and on our drive back home to New York City that evening. After that, we would talk about it with Tai Chi friends, as there was something pretty special about the world in reverse and these incredible moments and contrasts.

This was Lou's world, and he relished any evidence of this revealing itself—"Down for you is up" [from "Pale Blue Eyes"], the yin and yang of martial arts, the tension of love, the kiss with a punch. From his song "What's Good" from *Magic and Loss*: "What good's a war without killing? What good is rain that falls up? What good's a disease that won't hurt you? Why, no good, I guess, no good at all."

I flew in from Montana on October 26, 2013, to visit Lou out in the Springs. He was lying down in the living room, resting, and he was alert and, from what I could tell, happy to see me come in. I was shot out of a cannon, being anxious and not sure of his condition. I had moved to Montana in July, and this was the first time I was going to see Lou in four months. We had been communicating, via email, text, or phone as he was in and out of the hospital that summer and fall.

The first thing I said to him was, "What can I do to help you?" His answer: "Don't ask me that now, Scotty," with a smile. We spent the next few hours talking about everything. Most conversations with Lou were expansive. He was in a great deal of pain that afternoon, and we were trying to make him as comfortable as possible. Late in the afternoon, Lou demanded that we take him to the saltwater pool to warm up and hopefully do Tai Chi. His personal assistant, Jim Cass, and I took Lou into the heated saltwater pool to do Ren's 21 Form. Once he got into the water, he was fortified, showing great strength and balance as he led me in the form. He did two perfectly balanced forms, and that gave him temporary relief. We went back into the living room, where he bundled up to get warm and took a nap. I waited for him to wake up before I left, and he called my name to come in. He looked at me and said, "Give me a kiss goodbye," which I did, telling him

I loved him, and then offered to help him get into his bedroom to rest. I said that I would be back the next day (Sunday), and bring Ren with me after our 9 a.m. class on Lafayette Street.

I understood from Laurie that Lou did his Tai Chi before he passed away that Sunday morning. Ren, Dan, Hal, and friends gathered at the house that evening at Laurie's request, to help Lou pass into his new life and his rebirth.

STEPHAN BERWICK

Martial arts instructor and performer

My earliest recollection of martial arts was from about eight or nine years old. It was when the first Hong Kong martial arts movie appeared in the United States, which ignited the Kung Fu movie craze. The film was called *Five Fingers of Death*. To this day, I still remember every bit of the movie. It just blew my mind. The central character had a special technique where he trained his hands a certain way, in an old toughening technique called Iron Palm. The film was about him being pushed so far that he had to use his Iron Palm and basically destroy everybody with it.

The movie was actually made in the late '60s, but it didn't come to the States until the early '70s. It had such an impact. I still remember how everything changed after that. Everybody wanted to do martial arts. And we're talking before Bruce Lee became famous. *Five Fingers of Death* hit the United States and that was it. That's all I wanted to do. And there were kids everywhere—cities, countryside, everywhere. Everyone wanted to be martial artists, mimicking the moves they learned from the movies. We were on the streets making believe we were martial arts masters. And it all started from *Five Fingers of Death*.

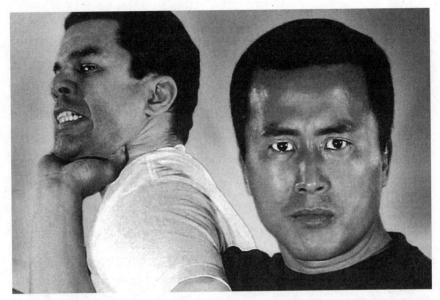

Stephan and Ren on the cover of Kung Fu Tai Chi *magazine in 2004*

I became a martial arts fanatic with a great dad who put me in the right direction with the arts. Books he got me pointed to Chinese martial arts, which at the time were hard to find, especially if you were not Chinese. My father made sure I saw a lot as a kid. He took me to the original, huge Aaron Banks events at Madison Square Garden to see a full gamut of martial arts. It was called the Oriental World of Self-Defense, which even appeared on national TV. Aaron Banks was a highlight of my childhood. It was the biggest annual event for me. We'd be there half the day. It was wild.

Lou's oldest martial arts friend, Bill O'Connor, mentioned that he and Lou went to the Aaron Banks exhibitions in the 1980s. My time going to the events was during the '70s. Aaron Banks was quite a character. And my dad used to love his events. Banks had a famous Jewish strongman perform—The Mighty Atom (Joe Greenstein)—who would bend things with his mouth and more. My father just loved this guy and thought he was the coolest dude ever. He'd come out wearing a yarmulke! And he was huge. He would do all this strongman stuff. And he was no youngster. He was in his sixties back then, with white hair and a long beard!

After training in Shotokan Karate, followed by Chinese martial arts under a teacher from Taiwan, I went to college in Boston and joined one of the best Chinese martial arts schools in the country at the time, the Chinese Wushu Research Institute, headed by a pioneer of Chinese martial arts and Tai Chi in the US, Bow Sim Mark, who is the mother of today's top action superstar in Asia, Donnie Yen. I spent so much time at her school, I dropped out of college, walking away from a full scholarship. All I wanted to do was train in martial arts.

She was amazing in that she was a pioneer of using traditional martial art as contemporary performance art. And she always advised me to get a strong foundation in the more external arts before moving to "internal" styles like Tai Chi. I heeded her advice. Little did I expect that my time there would take me to China with her son, as one of the first two Americans to train with China's top martial arts champion (Zhao Changjun) and coach (Bai Wenxian) in Xi'an. That was followed by working as an early Western martial arts film actor with Donnie, under the famed director Yuen Woo-ping, in Hong Kong.

After my training in China and martial arts film career in Hong Kong, I returned to New York to finish college. My older sister, a film costume designer who lived within Brooklyn's emerging art scene back then, suggested I get involved in film or other performance things. Through the grapevine she started, I was contacted by the musician and activist Fred Ho. He was just beginning to do stagings of his new martial arts operas in New York City, telling Chinese and African American stories. He was influenced by David Henry Hwang's *The Dance and the Railroad*, a musical that employed martial arts, which my father took me to see years before at Joseph Papp's Public

Theater. I'd heard of Ho's activism in Boston, but I didn't know much about him as a stalwart in jazz. When I met him, the first thing he talked about was how much Bow Sim Mark had inspired him to use Chinese martial arts as performance art. I was so impressed by that. He asked, "Would you be willing to work with me? I'm about to launch single-act stagings, but I need the right kind of martial arts choreography to prove the concept." Without hesitation, I said yes. The first performance took place at Avery Fisher Hall, featuring the Asian American performance group Slant.

While working with Ho, I heard about a Chen family–trained Tai Chi instructor teaching in New York, who turned out to be Ren. My dad and I went to his first teaching locale at a Chinese martial arts school in Flushing. He had been teaching for about six months. Greg Pinney was there, and José Figueroa joined just before I did. I saw immediately that it was the real deal. I saw Ren as a very professional, very intense and polished, serious training martial artist. For Tai Chi, that was rare to see in the United States.

I was drawn to his professionalism, discipline, and authenticity, which fortified his teaching and fueled the growth of his classes and recognition. As his group grew, Ren started to, I guess you could say, flex his muscles. He began saying that he had to do more with his Tai Chi, including film work. So of course I brought Donnie to one of Ren's classes. Donnie spent half the day with us. At the time, Donnie was becoming a big star in Asia. Ren was of course excited and performed Xin Jia (New Frame, of Chen Tai Chi) for Donnie in front of the class. Donnie saw Ren very much the way I saw him, as the serious, authentic, professional Tai Chi man. There was always something pure about that.

As Ren's student base grew, he began to attract celebrities and other prominent personalities to his classes. The first was actor Scott Glenn, a longtime martial artist. I discussed with Glenn how best to promote Ren and Chen Tai Chi. I then ramped up my writing about Ren and Chen Tai Chi in the martial arts press. He then got featured in more martial arts magazines including once being on the covers of *Inside Kung-Fu* and *Kung Fu Tai Chi* magazines simultaneously! By the early 2000s, Ren was the man for Tai Chi in New York. Lou joined at this time.

When Ren told me he was teaching Lou, I didn't know to what extent. I was not aware of Lou's passion for this. I first met him in 2003 at one of the nation's biggest martial arts events held in California. Our meeting was not just a dinner or a hello at a party. It was the three of us spending four days together at this giant martial arts event. Ren arranged for us to be interviewed by *Kung Fu Tai Chi* magazine there, which was a commemoration of their fifteenth anniversary. Back then the publication was becoming the top English-language magazine for traditional Chinese martial arts. That was the first time Lou appeared in the martial arts press.

My first hour with him, I felt, *This man is completely into this stuff*. I did not expect him to be so open and in love with martial arts. I thought he was maybe doing it just for health, meditation, or as an easygoing fun thing. But he was into all of it. And he just loved martial artists. Lou and Ren were just getting to know each other. But they knew that was it for them. Lou was already committed to Ren, and Ren told me, "This guy, this is an amazing person." So the bond was there from the beginning.

That weekend cemented what we thought would be a good vision for Ren. And part of that, or the nucleus of it, was that Ren had to perform with Lou on a wider scale, because we knew that as long as Ren is focused on doing what he does best, much could happen. And Ren was open to performing onstage with Lou. Lou felt something was there, something could happen with that. From the beginning, he insisted that we had to get Ren out there more.

Lou didn't have depth in Chen Tai Chi yet. A lot of what he saw in Ren is really what Chen Tai Chi is all about. But he was soaking it up rapidly. Whenever I visited New York from my new home in DC, I would go to Lou's place on 11th Street with my computers to work from there while Lou and Ren trained on the roof. I would join them after. That was the routine. So as Lou advanced, we all got closer.

Lou would also come to DC when I hosted Ren for seminars. We had so much fun together, sharing the martial arts passion and strategizing about how best to promote Ren and Chen Tai Chi more widely. Lou would often call me with, "Hey, Steph, what does this mean?" Or, "Why is Ren saying that?" Or, "I read this—what is it about?" He would call about once a month to discuss martial arts or Ren, bonding us further.

Once Lou called me about Ren after returning from a European tour. They bickered about something, and Lou called me up to talk about it. I remember trying my best to explain to Lou that Ren comes from good people. He lived a kind of street-hood lifestyle when he was training under Chen Xiaowang in Zhengzhou, China. I told him that while Ren has a tough guy thing about him, I reminded Lou that Ren comes from a nice family, whom I know personally. Lou said, "All right. I get it. I just want to be sure, because if we're going to keep doing anything else, I just want to be sure what's up." Lou, at times, wasn't at his best either. Yet Ren never complained to me about Lou, even at times when Lou questioned me about Ren, frustrated dealing with an old-school Chinese martial arts teacher.

But Lou was so comfortable in a solid martial arts group or brotherhood. He just loved being around tough guys, especially tough guys who were artists, who actually had something else to offer or were about something more. So when he met Ren, it stirred something in him.

Ren always said to me, "We have to do something together. You were in martial arts movies," and I usually responded lukewarm. Having been in martial arts films, I was quite realistic about how hard it is to make action films. But he encouraged me to write something, to come up with an idea for a film. Lou was open to it, so I wrote a concept that I had years ago, with specific selections of Lou's music added. We presented it to Lou late one night at a Korean restaurant in Manhattan. He said, "Yeah, I get this. I think there's something here. We can do something." He gave me extraordinary permission to use whatever of his music I wanted. A short time later, we made the short film *Final Weapon*—a film that was challenging to make yet captured something very special.

The obscure Maya Deren film from 1948, *Meditation on Violence*, was very important to Lou. He spoke to me about it when we first met. I'd heard of the film but didn't know who Deren was. It was like a mystery to us. Lou thought there was something deep and hypnotic about the film. Deren filmed a young Chinese American stage and film actor, who decades later acted in the famous film *Big Trouble in Little China* in the '80s. I had no idea that he was a well-qualified martial artist, because he came up during a time when Chinese martial arts were kept quiet within the Chinese community. They barely or rarely taught people outside their community. But he was a stage performer and apparently knew Deren, who was a film artist. What they created was an early, compelling example of traditional Chinese martial art as modern performance art. When we did *Final Weapon*, Deren's film was a big topic of discussion.

Final Weapon gave Lou the same feeling he got when he watched the Maya Deren piece. He was delighted with how I handled his music in the film. Lou included the film in an exhibit of his photography in Lisbon, where he described how the piece captured the power and magic of Tai Chi. He took my breath away when he told me, "My music finally has a home in *Final Weapon*."

Without Lou's or Ren's knowledge, I submitted the film to the New Filmmakers series at Jonas Mekas's Anthology Film Archives. I was thrilled when it got accepted. After the screening and Q&A, Lou, Jonas, and I had a private discussion about the film. Jonas said to me, "There's a piece of magic captured here that even for Lou is maybe hard to capture, and your film grabs it. If you guys can do more with it, you must." Hearing that from the film artist and critic that Mekas was stunned me. And Lou was right there by my side for that.

Lou truly enjoyed being around martial artists. I think it filled something he was missing. Not everybody knew who he was, but he was connected to a top dog in that world. When Lou was around Ren and his martial art brothers and sisters, he felt strong. Maybe he felt protected or secure. I'll even say he felt kind of cool.

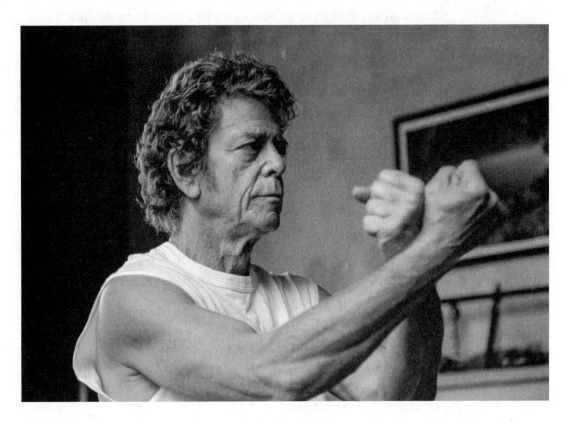

Lou in Chen Tai Chi double fists

AFTERWORD

LAURIE ANDERSON

I have to say, it's strange and wonderful to collaborate with someone who's been dead for almost ten years. We're working in Lou's afterlife now, trying to imagine what he would do as the author of this book and how to keep trying to push his ideas and energy forward. Along with the joy and guesswork, it's also been wrenching. I was with Lou for twenty-one years. He was my partner and best friend. Like with many couples, when Lou died, part of me died too, and sometimes it's hard to remember the way things actually were.

Lou's work ethic was truly powerful. Yet you never saw him working. He looked like he was doing absolutely nothing, and then suddenly he had just finished an opera with Bob Wilson. Or he had just written every song of a whole new record. He would never say, "Oh, I'm having a really hard time with this or that." He would just do it and it was suddenly there.

When I first met Lou in 1992, he was in a surge of creativity. He was involved in a million different things—movies, tours, PR, people, and all sorts of side projects. It was a whirlwind. We were both busy with tours and recording. It was in the midst of all this that I first went to Eagle Claw class with him. Bill O'Connor was also in the class, and they talked about being intimidated by the athleticism. Somebody comes at you, and you're supposed to just somersault away. Now, who can actually do a handspring while escaping? In the frequent open-class demos, Lou and Bill went leaping around in circles. It was like going to the circus. I'd never seen people do stuff like that. I think that theatricality was a big attraction for both of them at the beginning. But Lou knew and loved operas and movies full of theatrical Tai Chi. I wasn't a Bruce Lee fan when I met Lou, but I became one. Watching Bruce Lee reminds me of how Lou would laugh his wild, crazy laugh, literally howling when Bruce came up with a brand-new move.

Lou also saw Tai Chi as a way to find calm balance and acceleration. I think another thing Lou noted about Bruce Lee was that he could be wound up and an instant later incredibly relaxed. This concept of being complex and "ready" made a big impression on Lou. He recognized this quality in Brando too—a highly stylized person on the outside and yet somehow completely at ease. This was the balance of power and grace he talked about. It's also the way Lou played his solo shows, with confidence and simplicity. No posing. It can take lifetimes to learn how to be relaxed and attentive at the same time.

Bill O'Connor pointed out that when Lou and Master Ren met years later, they recognized the performer in each other. They both loved to perform and had their own original and well-developed theatricality and styles. And they brought that out in each other. They were also capable of being raucous ten-year-olds. I remember many times coming home and watching them running through the house literally shrieking with laughter and trying to knock each other over.

Of course it's tempting to try to guess what draws people to Tai Chi and how it helps them and who they'd be without it. Lou's reputation as a difficult and angry person was part of his rock star legend. But in my opinion, it was his honesty that made people nervous. Lou didn't have the usual filters. He said what he thought. And sometimes that included undisguised anger. In general, as editors, we've tried to be very careful about speculating what effects Tai Chi has on people's lives. We agreed that often we don't even understand our own motives so guessing what motivates other people starts to sound like amateur shrinking. Lou's career was full of journalists eager to psychoanalyze him based on his lyrics, no matter how many times he insisted, "It's called writing!" That said, I got to see firsthand how Lou related to Tai Chi, which was a complex mix of effort, dependence, and inspiration. It was the same energy and ardor that propelled Lou as an artist.

Lou's approach to Tai Chi was like everything else: he wanted the best, and he was willing to put a lot of time into researching computers, suitcases, microphones, or raincoats. "I'm going to find the best Tai Chi teacher. I'm going to find the best weapons. I'm going to find the best form. Then I'm going to work at it." And then there was Lou's enthusiasm and his pride in his progress. "Feel my back! I didn't have that last week." "Feel my calf!" "Can you believe that?" Even when he couldn't walk because of his toe, he would walk anyway.

Lou's health problems began in the mid-'90s. "I know I'm going to die of liver cancer," he would say. But every day of his struggle with diabetes and hepatitis, he did extensive research on treatments. He became a proactive expert. Then he would do everything in his power—diet, exercise, experimental treatments—to stay in control of his health. This was his approach to life in general. If you don't like it, don't sit around trying to analyze why you don't like it. Fix it!

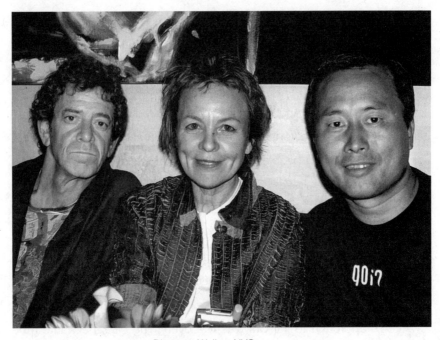

Dinner at Wallse, NYC

Lou loved to study Tai Chi—its philosophies, principles, and history. I inherited his large collection of eclectic and esoteric Tai Chi books. Lou was a great teacher, although he wouldn't have said that about himself. A lot of people have told me that they were able to learn from Lou because "He saw that I couldn't do it, and he broke it down for me." Lou liked to break things down. His own names for parts of the form, like Delivering the Pizza, became ways for people to relate to the moves with a sense of humor. His approach to Tai Chi was an elegant and original combination of loose, playful, rigorous, and respectfully traditional. Trying to master Tai Chi was at the top of his list. There were many mornings in my life with Lou when we were just waking up and it was then that we often talked about what we really wanted in life. These talks would ramble on for an hour or so. The lists of things changed over the years. What didn't shift for Lou was that at the top of all his lists was magic. He wanted to find magic. Tai Chi and music were the ways he looked for magic.

For Lou, doing Tai Chi wasn't only about his physical strength. Even when he could do it physically, he would say, "I'm doing it in my mind." "What do you mean you're doing it in your mind?" I'd say. "Are you picturing the moves?" "Yeah, I just picture them and then I feel them," he'd say. He could actually feel chi. He could pinpoint it, describe it, and trace the way it moved through his body. This was a mind-boggling teaching for me.

Sometimes he would demonstrate chi by passing one hand over the other, as in some of the moves in the 19 Form when the hands briefly describe a sphere. When I felt that for the first time, I was electrified. I was holding a ball of unbelievably powerful energy and realizing that it could move through me and that this is also what I was made of. Lou understood this intuitively.

After he died, I spent a lot of time talking with his friends Bill O'Connor and Hsia-Jung Chang. They had often met with Lou and talked about many of the more esoteric aspects of martial arts. They called these meetings the Seven Stars Club. I felt like I was given a glimpse into the secret heart of martial arts. Trying to understand this has become one of my motivations for studying.

Take me for what I am
a star newly emerging
long simmering explodes
inside the self is reeling.

Lou's lyrics sometimes seemed like codes. But the word "reeling" in the song "Set the Twilight Reeling" always reminded me of Tai Chi Silk

Reeling—one of the basic forms. And it's also about how to understand yourself as an energetic presence that continually unfolds.

In the last six years of his life, when he was studying every single day with Master Ren, the work ethic he'd applied to his music and writing was poured into Tai Chi. I remember the day he said, "The only thing I want to do now is Tai Chi." As he grew older and faced many health problems and increasing pain, he became even more aware of how profoundly the body and mind change. He often pointed out that we live in a country where people laugh at you when you're old. He was always quoting the familiar adage "Old age is not for sissies!" We were both very aware of the toll that age took on people, and we made note of how they dealt with it, some sinking into worse and worse moods and losing interest in life. Lou made a celebratory film called *Red Shirley* about his radical, hilarious, and badass cousin Shirley, who lived to be more than 100. Several people we interviewed for this book talked about how Tai Chi can help you in your old age. Lou was a super-cool young guy, but he was also a grand old man who had the funniest, most raucous sense of humor. And there was a grandeur about him, a steadiness and a magnificence that many old people simply do not have.

Lou also saw Tai Chi as a moving meditation, which you can hear in "Move Your Heart" and "Find Your Note" from *Hudson River Wind Meditations,* the pieces that Lou wrote for people to practice to. Lou was a committed meditator and a student of Yongey Mingyur Rinpoche. Together we spent a lot of time with our teacher, who helped both of us to strike a balance between dignity and vulnerability. I saw firsthand that it was Lou's meditation practice that made it possible for him to manage the incredible pain of his cancer and to face his death with equanimity.

One of the things that's hard to show in a book is sense of humor. Lou was the funniest guy I ever met. He was also the goofiest. When I get depressed or miss him too much, I think of Lou's goofy dancing. He would do dances for me that made me choke, I was laughing so hard. He counted on other people's sense of humor too and teased people a lot. Even when he was dying, he teased Charlie, his surgeon. "Charlie, you're getting so fat!" he'd say when he was being examined.

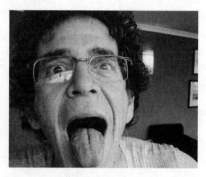

"You need to do some Tai Chi." Lou died on a Sunday. For the next forty-nine days we observed the traditional rituals associated with the Bardo, the Tibetan forty-nine-day period after death. Lou was familiar with this practice of honoring and supporting the transition from one form of consciousness to another. Each Sunday we did an event that featured different

Lou having fun practicing Tai Chi, Scotland

aspects of his life: friendship, design and photography, Tai Chi, music and meditation. Since Lou died, we have organized his extensive archive, which is now in the New York Public Library for the Performing Arts. We continue to do Lou Reed International Tai Chi Day as well as release an ongoing series of records and books.

Lou's two best friends, Hal Willner, his producer, and his Tai Chi brother Bill O'Connor, died while we've been working on this book. I've been think-ing of Lou's song "Sunday Morning," a song that feels like true Tai Chi to me. "Watch out, the world's behind you!" It reminds me of the way Master Ren begins practice sessions with the instruction, "Listen behind you."

And today I'm looking at the picture of Lou that hangs over my fire-place. He's looking out of the corner of his eye with the sweetest sadness you can possibly imagine. He's not fooling himself. Fortunately, I know there are a million other sides—he was capable of having a lot of joy and fun. Since his death, I think of him every day. I was in awe of the way he could combine dignity and sadness. He has somehow become my main teacher and the guardian angel I was always looking for.

Lou knew how to cry. He was the only man I ever met who could cry with innocence and passion. It's why I fell in love with him. He was, and continues to be, a gigantic person, and in the process of making this book, reading his words as well as the words of his friends, we as editors have gotten to know him all over again. When I miss him most, I think of the song he wrote for me when we got married called "The Power of the Heart."

You look for sun and I look for rain
We're different people, we're not the same
The power of the sun

I looked for treetops, you looked for caps
Above the water, where the waves snap back
I flew around the world to bring you back
Ah, the power of the heart

. . .

You know me I like to dream a lot
Of what there is and what there's not
But mainly I dream of you a lot
The power of your heart
The power of the heart

—LAURIE ANDERSON
Artist and Lou's partner for twenty-one years

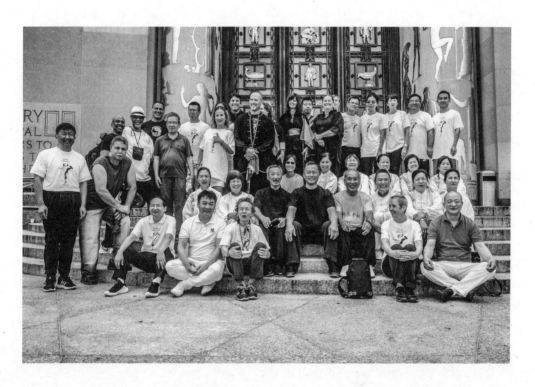

First annual Lou Reed International Tai Chi Day in Brooklyn, New York, 2019

IMAGE CREDITS

Page i: Lou Doing Tai Chi in the Afterlife, *Ramuntcho Matta, watercolor, 2016*

Page vii: Daily practice on the roof overlooking the Hudson River, Ren GuangYi

Page 310: Ren GuangYi's hand from Tai Chi's classic Single Whip technique, Lou Reed

Pages x, 8, 16, 100, 103, 109, 120, 127, 130, 155, 224, 247 (top), 260, 265, 268, 270, 271, 274, 280, 285, 298, photography insert 1–3: Ren GuangYi. Pages 2, 19, 23, 149, 167, 242, 259 (top): Mark McGauley. Pages 5, 67, 99, 105, 122, 123, 128, 129, 146, 150, 165, 168, 169, 186, 203 (top), 245, 279, 310: Lou Reed. Pages 25, 30: Ramuntcho Matta. Pages 39, 307: Daniel Efram. Pages 41, 42, 53, 54, 114, 181, 238: © Mick Rock. Page 47: © Frans Schellekens/Redferns/Getty Images. Pages 48, 81, 166, 200, 223: Amy-Beth McNeely. Page 57: Sharyn Felder. Page 61: *Inside Kung Fu*, 1982; www.insidekungfulive.com. Page 64: Music Division, the New York Public Library for the Performing Arts. Pages 66, 282: Jim Cass. Page 69: *New York Magazine*, September 15, 1986; photo: Lawrence Ivy. Page 73: Courtesy of Lenny Aaron. Page 79: Davide de Blasio. Page 89: © WENN Rights Ltd/Alamy Stock Photo. Page 91: Rob Verhorst/Redferns/Getty Images. Page 115: *The New Yorker*, 1996; illustration by Steve Brodner. Page 118: Courtesy of Iggy Pop. Pages 141, 145, 192, 229: Guido Harari. Page 154: Courtesy of Tergar. Page 156: Mingyur Rinpoche. Pages 175, 253: Dave Pabarcus. Page 178: *Meditation on Violence*, 16mm film by Maya Deren; © Tavia Ito, courtesy of Re:Voir. Page 182: *Fusion*, courtesy of Don Fleming. Pages 187, 188: Mark Seliger. Page 195: Julian Schnabel. Page 196: Sybill Schneider/Ullstein Bild/Getty Images. Page 203 (bottom): Eugene Gologursky/Getty Images. Page 206: © UPI/Alamy Stock Photo. Page 208: © Anton Corbijn. Page 209: Yvette Figueroa. Page 212: © 1993 Road Movies—Tobis Filmkunst; courtesy of Wim Wenders Stiftung. Pages 214, 256, photography insert 6–7: Portrait by Timothy Greenfield-Sanders. Pages 226, 302, 305: Scott Richman. Page 227: Bill Berger. Page 240: Courtesy of Worldwide Pants Inc. Page 247 (bottom): Jonathan Miller. Page 248 (bottom): Published by YMAA 2018. Page 258: © Jim Dyson/Getty Images. Page 259 (bottom): Daniel Boud. Page 291: Martin von Haselberg. Photography insert pages 4–5: Courtesy of *Kung Fu Tai Chi*.

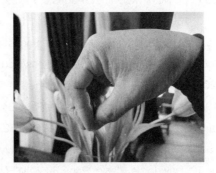

The editors would like to dedicate
The Art of the Straight Line
to Hal Willner, Bill O'Connor, and Mick Rock, all of
whom died while we were making this book.